OWEN HUNTER

The Men's Health Guide After 50

Contents

INTRODUCTION	1
CHAPTER 1	5
CHAPTER 2	13
CHAPTER 3	21
CHAPTER 4	32
CHAPTER 5	44
CHAPTER 6	53
CHAPTER 7	63
CHAPTER 8	72
CHAPTER 9	81
CHAPTER 10	91
CHAPTER 11	102
CHAPTER 12	111
CHAPTER 13	120
CHAPTER 14	130
CONCLUSION	139

INTRODUCTION

As the saying goes, "age is just a number." However, for many men, the transition into the second half of life can present a unique set of health challenges that require a proactive and comprehensive approach. The golden years are meant to be cherished, not plagued by preventable medical issues or a diminished quality of life. With the right knowledge, tools, and mindset, men can not only maintain their health and vitality well into their 50s, 60s, and beyond, but also discover newfound opportunities for growth, adventure, and fulfillment.

This book, "The Men's Health Guide After 50," is your roadmap to navigating the physical, mental, and emotional aspects of aging gracefully. Whether you are approaching your 50th birthday or are well into your retirement years, the advice and strategies outlined in these pages will empower you to take charge of your health, enhance your well-being, and thrive in the next chapter of your life.

The Changing Landscape of Men's Health

As men grow older, their healthcare needs and priorities often shift. Gone are the days of youthful invincibility, where minor aches and pains were easily brushed aside. Instead, men must now contend with a gradual yet steady decline in various physiological functions, ranging from cardiovascular health to cognitive abilities. The risk of developing chronic conditions, such as heart disease, diabetes, and certain types of cancer, also increases with age.

Compounding these physical changes are the emotional and psychological challenges that can arise later in life. The transition to retirement, the loss of loved ones, and the evolving dynamics within personal relationships can all contribute to feelings of isolation, depression, and anxiety. Maintaining a sense of purpose, social connection, and emotional well-being becomes increasingly critical as men navigate the uncharted waters of midlife and beyond.

The good news is that with the right approach, men can not only manage the effects of aging but also thrive in their later years. By proactively addressing health concerns, adopting healthy lifestyle habits, and cultivating a positive mindset, men can redefine what it means to grow older and reclaim their vitality.

A Holistic Approach to Men's Health After 50

This book takes a comprehensive and holistic approach to men's health, covering a wide range of topics that are essential for maintaining optimal well-being in the second half of life. From preventive screenings and cardiovascular health to hormonal changes, cognitive function, and sexual health, each chapter delves deep into the unique challenges faced by men and provides practical, evidence-based solutions.

Throughout the book, you will find a wealth of information to help you navigate the complex and ever-evolving landscape of healthcare. We'll explore the importance of regular check-ups, age-appropriate screening tests, and effective management strategies for common age-related conditions. Additionally, we'll address the often-overlooked mental and emotional aspects of aging, providing guidance on stress management, sleep optimization, and cultivating a fulfilling retirement.

One of the key pillars of this book is the emphasis on proactive and preventive measures. Rather than waiting for health problems to arise, we'll empower you to take a proactive stance, implementing lifestyle changes and incorporating proven strategies to maintain your well-being. By taking charge of your health today, you can significantly reduce the risk of chronic diseases, improve your quality of life, and set the stage for a vibrant and fulfilling future.

The Power of Positive Aging

Underlying the practical advice and medical guidance in this book is a fundamental belief: that growing older can be a time of renewal, growth, and endless possibilities. Too often, men are bombarded with the negative stereotypes and societal perceptions of aging, leading them to view their later years with dread and resignation. However, we firmly believe that the second half of life can be the most rewarding and fulfilling stage yet.

Throughout the book, we'll explore the importance of cultivating a positive mindset and embracing the unique opportunities that come with aging. Whether it's discovering new hobbies, rekindling relationships, or embarking on long-awaited adventures, men have the power to redefine their later years and create a life that is truly meaningful and satisfying.

By focusing on self-care, personal growth, and a sense of purpose, you can not only manage the physical and emotional challenges of aging but also unlock a newfound sense of vitality, confidence, and joie de vivre. This book will serve as your guide, empowering you to take control of your health, embrace the gifts of aging, and live your best life after 50.

A Call to Action

As you embark on this journey, remember that your health and well-being are not mere afterthoughts or something to be addressed only when problems arise. They are the foundation upon which you can build a fulfilling, rewarding, and adventurous life in your later years.

By reading this book and implementing the strategies and advice within, you are making a powerful investment in your future. You are taking a proactive step towards protecting your physical, mental, and emotional health, ensuring that you can enjoy the second half of your life to the fullest.

So, let's get started. The path to vibrant, healthy, and purposeful aging begins now. Embrace the challenge, trust the process, and get ready to embark on an extraordinary new chapter of your life.

CHAPTER 1

Embracing the Journey After 50

As the old adage goes, "with age comes wisdom." While there is undoubtedly truth to this sentiment, the reality is that growing older also brings with it a unique set of health challenges and considerations. For men embarking on the second half of their lives, navigating the physical, mental, and emotional changes can feel daunting and overwhelming at times.

However, it is important to remember that the journey of aging is not one to be feared, but rather embraced with a sense of purpose, resilience, and optimism. By understanding the unique health needs of men over 50 and developing a proactive mindset, you can not only manage the effects of aging but also unlock new opportunities for growth, fulfillment, and an enhanced quality of life.

In this chapter, we will explore the fundamental aspects of embracing the journey after 50, delving into the specific health challenges you may face and the strategies to address them. We will also discuss the importance of cultivating a positive mindset and a holistic approach to your well-being, laying the groundwork for the comprehensive guidance that will be provided throughout this book.

Understanding the Unique Health Challenges of Aging

As men transition into their 50s, 60s, and beyond, their bodies and overall health undergo a gradual, yet significant, transformation. These changes, while natural and inevitable, can nonetheless be daunting and require a keen understanding to effectively manage them.

One of the primary concerns that often arises with age is the decline in various physiological functions. This can manifest in a variety of ways, such as:

1. Cardiovascular health: As men grow older, the risk of developing heart disease, high blood pressure, and other cardiovascular conditions increases. The gradual stiffening of blood vessels, coupled with the buildup of plaque, can compromise the heart's ability to pump blood efficiently, leading to a heightened risk of heart attacks, strokes, and other life-threatening events.

2. Musculoskeletal health: The aging process can also take a toll on the musculoskeletal system, leading to a gradual loss of bone density, muscle mass, and flexibility. This can contribute to an increased risk of fractures, joint pain, and mobility issues, potentially limiting an individual's physical independence and quality of life.

3. Hormonal changes: Another significant health consideration for men after 50 is the decline in testosterone production. This hormonal shift can have far-reaching effects, including changes in sexual function, mood, energy levels, and overall body composition.

4. Cognitive function: As the brain ages, men may experience a gradual decline in cognitive abilities, such as memory, processing speed, and problem-solving skills. While mild cognitive changes are a normal part of aging, more significant impairments, such as those associated with Alzheimer's disease or other forms of dementia, can have a profound impact on an individual's daily life and independence.

5. Urological health: Men's urological health also becomes an increasing concern as they grow older. Issues such as an enlarged prostate, incontinence, and erectile dysfunction can significantly impact quality of life and overall well-being.

These are just a few of the many health challenges that men may face as they navigate the later stages of life. It is important to note that the specific effects and timelines of these changes can vary greatly from individual to individual, influenced by factors such as genetics, lifestyle habits, and overall health status.

Developing a Positive Mindset for Lifelong Wellness

While the health challenges associated with aging may seem daunting, it is crucial to approach this journey with a positive and proactive mindset. Embracing the process of aging, rather than dreading it, can make all the difference in your ability to maintain your well-being and thrive in the years to come.

1. Redefining the Aging Narrative

   One of the first steps in cultivating a positive mindset is to challenge the negative stereotypes and societal perceptions that often surround aging. Instead of viewing growing older as a time of decline and diminished capabilities, strive to redefine the narrative and see it as an opportunity for growth, wisdom, and newfound experiences.

It is important to remember that aging is a natural and inevitable process, not a disease to be feared. By shifting your perspective and focusing on the potential that lies ahead, you can unlock a renewed sense of purpose, vitality, and enthusiasm for the next chapter of your life.

2. Celebrating Milestones and Achievements

   As you navigate the journey of aging, take the time to celebrate your milestones and achievements, both big and small. Whether it's reaching a significant birthday, achieving a personal goal, or simply enjoying a fulfilling day, acknowledging these moments can foster a deep sense of gratitude and appreciation for the life you have lived.

Celebrating your accomplishments, no matter how seemingly ordinary, can help reinforce the idea that your life is a tapestry of rich experiences and meaningful contributions. This, in turn, can instill a greater sense of self-worth and confidence as you move forward.

3. Embracing Lifelong Learning

One of the hallmarks of a positive mindset is a genuine curiosity and openness to learning throughout one's life. As men enter the second half of their lives, they have the unique opportunity to explore new hobbies, acquire new skills, and engage in intellectual pursuits that may have been put on the backburner during their younger, busier years.

By embracing the concept of lifelong learning, you can keep your mind sharp, stimulate your creativity, and discover new passions that can enrich your life. Whether it's taking a cooking class, learning a new language, or delving into a subject that has always intrigued you, the act of continuous learning can foster a sense of fulfillment, purpose, and personal growth.

4. Prioritizing Self-Care and Well-Being

Maintaining a positive mindset is not just about changing your perspective; it also requires a commitment to prioritizing your overall well-being. This means making deliberate choices to engage in self-care practices that nourish your physical, mental, and emotional health.

This can include regular exercise, a balanced and nutritious diet, adequate sleep, stress management techniques, and engaging in activities that bring you joy and relaxation. By prioritizing your own needs and well-being, you can build a strong foundation for a healthier, more resilient, and more fulfilling later life.

5. Fostering Meaningful Connections

As men age, the importance of maintaining and cultivating meaningful social connections becomes increasingly vital. Strong relationships with family, friends, and community can provide a sense of belonging, support, and purpose, all of which are essential for emotional well-being and overall quality of life.

Whether it's reconnecting with old friends, joining a local club or organization, or nurturing your family ties, make a conscious effort to prioritize these meaningful connections. Engaging in social activities, sharing experiences, and leaning on your support system can help combat feelings of isolation and loneliness, which can often accompany the aging process.

Embracing the Holistic Approach to Men's Health

While the physical, mental, and emotional changes associated with aging can be daunting, it is important to remember that your health and well-being are interconnected. A holistic approach that addresses the various facets of your life is essential for maintaining optimal health and a high quality of life in your later years.

1. Preventive Care and Regular Check-ups

One of the cornerstones of a holistic approach to men's health after 50 is a focus on preventive care and regular check-ups. By staying proactive and diligent with your healthcare, you can identify potential issues early on and take the necessary steps to manage or even prevent them.

This includes scheduling regular physical examinations, obtaining age-appropriate screening tests (such as prostate exams, cancer screenings, and cardiovascular assessments), and maintaining open communication with your healthcare providers. Preventive care not only helps to catch problems in their early stages but also empowers you to take an active role in safeguarding your long-term well-being.

2. Lifestyle Modifications and Healthy Habits

In addition to preventive care, adopting a healthy lifestyle and incorporating sustainable habits is crucial for maintaining your overall health and vitality. This can include:

- Engaging in regular physical activity, such as strength training, cardiovascular exercise, and flexibility-enhancing activities
  - Consuming a balanced, nutrient-dense diet that supports your changing nutritional needs
  - Managing stress through relaxation techniques, mindfulness practices, and work-life balance
  - Prioritizing quality sleep and maintaining a consistent sleep schedule
  - Avoiding or moderating the use of tobacco, alcohol, and other substances that can negatively impact your health

By making these lifestyle modifications and cultivating healthy habits, you can proactively address many of the age-related health challenges and optimize your physical, mental, and emotional well-being.

3. Emotional and Mental Health Considerations

While physical health is undoubtedly important, it is equally crucial to address the emotional and mental health aspects of aging. The transition into the later stages of life can bring about significant changes and challenges, such as retirement, the loss of loved ones, and the evolution of personal relationships.

To maintain a healthy and balanced perspective, it is essential to prioritize your emotional well-being. This may involve seeking support from mental health professionals, engaging in stress management techniques, and fostering a strong support network of family and friends. By addressing your emotional and mental health needs, you can better navigate the ups and downs of aging and cultivate a greater sense of resilience and fulfillment.

4. Integrated Healthcare Approach

Embracing a holistic approach to your health also means adopting an integrated healthcare model that considers the various aspects of your well-being. This may involve collaborating with a team of healthcare providers, including your primary care physician, specialists (such as cardiologists, urologists, or geriatric specialists), mental health professionals, and other allied healthcare practitioners.

By working closely with this integrated team, you can ensure that your unique health needs are addressed in a comprehensive and coordinated manner. This collaborative approach can help you make more informed decisions, identify potential risk factors, and develop a personalized plan of action that optimizes your overall health and quality of life.

Embarking on the Journey of Vibrant Aging

As you embark on the journey of aging after 50, remember that this is not simply a time of decline, but rather an opportunity to redefine your life and unlock new possibilities. By embracing a positive mindset, addressing the unique health challenges you may face, and adopting a holistic approach to your well-being, you can navigate this chapter of your life with confidence, resilience, and a renewed sense of purpose.

The road ahead may have its twists and turns, but with the right mindset, tools, and support, you can overcome obstacles, maintain your independence, and create a fulfilling and rewarding later life. Embrace the journey, celebrate the milestones, and trust that the wisdom and experiences you've gained over the years will be your greatest assets as you continue to evolve and thrive.

Remember, the best is yet to come. Let's embark on this adventure together, and make the most of the years that lie ahead.

CHAPTER 2

Mastering Preventive Health Screenings

As men approach their 50s and beyond, the importance of proactive and preventive healthcare becomes increasingly critical. Gone are the days when a brief annual check-up or occasional doctor's visit was enough to maintain good health. The shifting landscape of men's health, coupled with the gradual physiological changes that come with aging, necessitates a more comprehensive and diligent approach to preventive care.

In this chapter, we will delve into the vital role of preventive health screenings and examinations in preserving your long-term well-being. We'll explore the key tests and assessments that every man over 50 should prioritize, the importance of early detection and intervention, and strategies for effectively navigating the healthcare system to ensure you receive the care you need.

The Significance of Preventive Health Screenings

Preventive health screenings are the cornerstone of maintaining optimal health and longevity. These targeted tests and examinations serve as early warning systems, allowing healthcare providers to identify potential issues before they escalate into more serious and potentially life-threatening conditions.

As men grow older, their risk for a wide range of health problems, from cardiovascular disease and cancer to cognitive decline and urological issues, increases significantly. Preventive screenings provide the opportunity to catch these concerns in their earliest stages, when they are often more treatable and manageable.

Consider the following examples:

1. Prostate Cancer Screening: Prostate cancer is one of the most common types of cancer among men, with the risk increasing dramatically after the age of 50. Regular prostate-specific antigen (PSA) tests and digital rectal examinations can help detect prostate cancer in its earliest, most treatable stages, ultimately improving outcomes and saving lives.

2. Colon Cancer Screening: Colorectal cancer is another prevalent concern for men as they age. Screening tests, such as colonoscopies, can identify precancerous polyps or early-stage cancers, allowing for timely intervention and potentially preventing the development of more advanced disease.

3. Cardiovascular Health Assessments: Regular check-ups that include blood pressure measurements, cholesterol tests, and other cardiovascular evaluations can help identify and manage conditions like hypertension, high cholesterol, and atherosclerosis before they lead to life-threatening events like heart attacks or strokes.

4. Cognitive Function Evaluations: As men age, they may experience subtle changes in cognitive function, such as memory lapses or difficulty with problem-solving. Comprehensive neuropsychological assessments can help detect the early signs of cognitive decline, enabling timely intervention and the implementation of strategies to maintain brain health.

By consistently engaging in preventive health screenings, men can take a proactive approach to their well-being, empowering themselves to make informed decisions, take appropriate actions, and ultimately enhance their quality of life as they grow older.

Understanding the Importance of Age-Appropriate Screenings

One of the key principles of effective preventive healthcare is the recognition that the specific screening tests and examinations required evolve as men progress through different stages of life. What may have been an appropriate set of screenings in your 40s may not be the same as what is recommended in your 60s or 70s.

This age-tailored approach to preventive care is crucial for several reasons:

1. Changing Risk Profiles: As men age, their risk profiles for various health conditions shift. Certain conditions, such as prostate cancer or cognitive decline, become more prevalent in the later stages of life, necessitating more targeted screening efforts.

2. Evolving Screening Guidelines: Medical organizations and healthcare authorities regularly review and update their recommendations for preventive screenings based on the latest research and evidence. Keeping up with these evolving guidelines ensures that you are receiving the most appropriate care for your current age and health status.

3. Personalized Needs: Each man's individual health history, genetic predispositions, and lifestyle factors can influence the specific screening tests that are most relevant and beneficial. A one-size-fits-all approach to preventive care may not be effective, and a more personalized approach is often required.

By understanding the importance of age-appropriate screenings and staying informed about the latest guidelines, you can work closely with your healthcare providers to develop a comprehensive preventive care plan that addresses your unique needs and concerns.

Navigating the Healthcare System Effectively

Navigating the complex and often-fragmented healthcare system can be a daunting task, particularly when it comes to ensuring that you receive the preventive care you need. However, by developing a proactive and strategic approach, you can overcome these challenges and ensure that your health remains a top priority.

1. Establishing a Relationship with a Primary Care Provider
   A primary care provider, such as a family medicine physician or an internist, serves as the cornerstone of your preventive healthcare journey. This healthcare professional will be responsible for coordinating your care, ordering necessary screenings, and providing personalized recommendations based on your age, health status, and risk factors.

When choosing a primary care provider, consider factors such as their experience, communication style, and commitment to preventive care. Establishing a long-term relationship with a trusted healthcare provider can facilitate more effective and personalized care over time.

2. Staying Informed About Screening Guidelines
   Keeping up with the latest recommendations for preventive health screenings is crucial. Medical organizations, such as the American Academy of Family Physicians, the U.S. Preventive Services Task Force, and disease-specific associations, regularly publish updated guidelines that outline the appropriate timing and frequency of various screening tests.

By educating yourself about these guidelines and discussing them with your primary care provider, you can ensure that your preventive care plan aligns with the most current and evidence-based recommendations.

3. Advocating for Your Healthcare Needs

As an active participant in your own healthcare, it is important to advocate for the preventive screenings and examinations that you believe are necessary. This may involve having open and honest discussions with your healthcare providers, expressing your concerns and preferences, and working collaboratively to develop a personalized preventive care plan.

Remember, you are the expert on your own health, and your input and involvement are essential in ensuring that you receive the highest quality of care. Don't be afraid to ask questions, seek second opinions, or request additional testing if you feel it is warranted.

4. Navigating Insurance and Financial Considerations

The financial aspects of healthcare can be a significant concern, especially when it comes to preventive screenings and examinations. It is important to understand your health insurance coverage, including the scope of preventive care benefits and any out-of-pocket costs associated with various tests and procedures.

If you encounter challenges or limitations with your insurance coverage, explore alternative options, such as community health programs, sliding-scale clinics, or financial assistance programs that may be available to help you access the necessary preventive care without compromising your financial well-being.

5. Maintaining Consistent Communication with Providers

Effective preventive healthcare requires ongoing communication and collaboration between you and your healthcare providers. Make it a priority to attend all scheduled appointments, follow up on test results, and discuss any changes in your health or concerns that arise.

By maintaining open and transparent communication, you can ensure that your healthcare providers have a comprehensive understanding of your overall well-being, enabling them to make informed decisions and adjust your preventive care plan as needed.

Putting Preventive Health Screenings into Practice

Now that we have explored the importance of preventive health screenings and the strategies for navigating the healthcare system, let's delve into the specific tests and examinations that every man over 50 should prioritize.

1. Cardiovascular Health Screenings

Maintaining cardiovascular health is a crucial aspect of preventive care for men as they age. Regular screenings should include:

- Blood pressure measurements: Monitor for hypertension, which can increase the risk of heart disease and stroke.
- Cholesterol tests: Identify and manage high levels of LDL (bad) cholesterol, which can contribute to the development of atherosclerosis.
- Electrocardiogram (ECG): Assess the electrical activity of the heart for any abnormalities.
- Stress tests: Evaluate the heart's performance during physical activity to detect potential issues.

2. Cancer Screening Tests

Early detection of cancer is paramount, and men over 50 should undergo the following screenings:

- Prostate cancer screening: Annual digital rectal exams and PSA (prostate-specific antigen) blood tests to detect prostate cancer in its earliest stages.
- Colorectal cancer screening: Colonoscopies or other screening methods to identify precancerous polyps or early-stage colorectal cancer.
- Lung cancer screening: Low-dose CT scans for individuals with a history of heavy smoking.
- Skin cancer screening: Regular skin examinations to detect any suspicious

moles or lesions.

3. Urological Health Assessments

As men age, their urological health becomes an increasingly important concern. Regular screenings should include:

- Prostate exam: Digital rectal examination and PSA blood test to assess prostate health and detect any abnormalities.
- Urinalysis: Analysis of urine samples to identify potential issues like urinary tract infections or signs of prostate enlargement.
- Erectile dysfunction evaluation: Assessment of sexual function and potential underlying causes.

4. Cognitive Function Evaluations

Maintaining cognitive health is crucial as men grow older. Preventive screenings in this area should consist of:

- Neuropsychological assessment: Comprehensive evaluation of memory, cognitive abilities, and overall brain function.
- Dementia screening: Tests to detect the early signs of cognitive decline or the onset of conditions like Alzheimer's disease.

5. Musculoskeletal Health Assessments

The aging process can take a toll on the musculoskeletal system, making regular screenings essential. These may include:

- Bone density scan (DEXA): Measure bone mineral density to detect the presence of osteoporosis or increased fracture risk.
- Joint examinations: Assessment of joint function, flexibility, and any signs of osteoarthritis or other degenerative conditions.

6. Metabolic and Endocrine Screenings

Maintaining a healthy metabolic and hormonal balance is crucial for overall well-being. Recommended screenings in this area include:

- Diabetes screening: Blood glucose tests to detect the presence of prediabetes or type 2 diabetes.
   - Thyroid function tests: Evaluation of thyroid hormone levels to identify any imbalances.
   - Testosterone assessment: Measurement of testosterone levels to identify any age-related decline or hormonal imbalances.

Remember, the specific screening schedule and frequency may vary based on your individual health history, risk factors, and any recommendations from your healthcare provider. It is essential to work closely with your primary care physician to develop a personalized preventive care plan that addresses your unique needs and concerns.

Embracing Preventive Healthcare for a Healthier Future

Preventive health screenings are not just a box to check off; they are a vital investment in your long-term well-being. By consistently engaging in these targeted assessments, you are taking proactive steps to safeguard your health, identify potential issues early, and empower yourself to make informed decisions about your care.

As you navigate the journey of aging, remember that preventive healthcare is not a one-time event, but rather a lifelong commitment. Stay informed, communicate openly with your healthcare providers, and be an active participant in the process. By doing so, you can ensure that you receive the tailored care you need to maintain optimal health and vitality in the years to come.

Embrace the power of preventive health screenings, and embark on a path towards a healthier, more fulfilling future. Your well-being is worth the investment, and the peace of mind it can provide is priceless.

CHAPTER 3

Optimizing Cardiovascular Health

As men transition into their 50s and beyond, maintaining a healthy cardiovascular system becomes increasingly crucial. The aging process brings with it a host of changes that can significantly impact the heart and the circulatory system, elevating the risk of life-threatening conditions such as heart disease, stroke, and hypertension.

In this chapter, we will delve into the fundamental aspects of cardiovascular health for men over 50. We'll explore the physiological changes that occur, the common cardiovascular conditions that men may face, and the essential strategies for preserving a healthy heart and blood vessels through diet, exercise, and effective management of risk factors.

Understanding the Aging Cardiovascular System

The human cardiovascular system is a remarkable and complex network of blood vessels, the heart, and other vital components that work together to deliver oxygen-rich blood throughout the body. However, as the body ages, this intricate system undergoes gradual yet significant changes that can compromise its overall efficiency and resilience.

1. Structural Changes in the Heart
   One of the primary changes that occur in the aging cardiovascular system

is the gradual stiffening and thickening of the heart muscle. This process, known as cardiac hypertrophy, can reduce the heart's ability to efficiently pump blood, leading to a decrease in cardiac output and an increase in the workload on the heart.

Additionally, the valves within the heart may also become stiffer and less flexible, further hindering the heart's ability to effectively circulate blood. These structural changes can contribute to the development of various cardiovascular conditions, such as diastolic dysfunction, aortic stenosis, and heart failure.

2. Vascular Alterations

As men grow older, their blood vessels, including the arteries and veins, also undergo significant changes. The walls of these vessels can become less elastic and more rigid, a condition known as arteriosclerosis. This loss of elasticity can lead to an increase in blood pressure, as the heart must work harder to push blood through the less flexible vessels.

Furthermore, the buildup of plaque within the arteries, a process called atherosclerosis, can restrict blood flow and increase the risk of life-threatening events like heart attacks and strokes. This gradual narrowing and hardening of the arteries can have far-reaching consequences for overall cardiovascular health.

3. Hormonal Changes

Another factor that can significantly impact cardiovascular health in men over 50 is the decline in testosterone production. As testosterone levels gradually decrease with age, this can contribute to changes in body composition, increased abdominal fat, and a heightened risk of developing conditions like metabolic syndrome and type 2 diabetes.

These hormonal shifts can have a cascading effect on the cardiovascular system, increasing the likelihood of developing hypertension, dyslipidemia (abnormal cholesterol and triglyceride levels), and other risk factors for heart disease.

Understanding these age-related changes in the cardiovascular system is the first step in developing an effective strategy for preserving heart health and preventing the onset of cardiovascular problems.

Common Cardiovascular Conditions in Men After 50

As men navigate the later stages of life, they face an increased risk of developing a variety of cardiovascular conditions. It is crucial to be aware of these common issues and take proactive steps to manage them effectively.

1. Coronary Artery Disease

Coronary artery disease, also known as ischemic heart disease, is one of the most prevalent cardiovascular conditions among men over 50. This condition is characterized by the buildup of plaque within the coronary arteries, which supply blood and oxygen to the heart muscle.

As the arteries become narrowed and blocked, the heart's ability to function efficiently is compromised, leading to symptoms such as chest pain (angina), shortness of breath, and an increased risk of heart attacks. Identifying and managing coronary artery disease through lifestyle modifications, medications, and potentially, interventional procedures, is crucial for maintaining cardiovascular health.

2. Hypertension (High Blood Pressure)

Hypertension, or high blood pressure, is another common cardiovascular concern for men in their later years. As the arteries become less elastic and the heart has to work harder to pump blood, the pressure within the blood vessels can rise to unhealthy levels.

Uncontrolled hypertension can significantly increase the risk of a wide range of cardiovascular problems, including heart attacks, strokes, and heart failure. Effectively managing hypertension through a combination of lifestyle changes, medication, and regular monitoring is essential for maintaining optimal cardiovascular health.

3. Heart Failure

Heart failure, a condition in which the heart is unable to pump blood effectively, is a growing concern for men as they age. This can be the result of various underlying factors, such as coronary artery disease, hypertension, or structural changes within the heart itself.

Symptoms of heart failure may include shortness of breath, fatigue, swelling in the legs and feet, and difficulty performing everyday activities. Proactive management of heart failure, often involving a combination of medication, lifestyle modifications, and potentially surgical interventions, is crucial for preserving heart function and quality of life.

4. Arrhythmias

Irregular heartbeats, or arrhythmias, are another common cardiovascular issue that can affect men over 50. These abnormal heart rhythms can range from harmless premature contractions to more serious conditions like atrial fibrillation, which can increase the risk of stroke and other complications.

Identifying and managing arrhythmias, often through the use of medications, medical devices, or even surgical procedures, is essential for maintaining a healthy and consistent heart rhythm.

5. Peripheral Artery Disease

Peripheral artery disease (PAD) is a condition in which the arteries that supply blood to the limbs, particularly the legs, become narrowed or blocked due to the buildup of plaque. This can lead to symptoms such as leg pain, cramping, or even gangrene, and can significantly increase the risk of cardiovascular events.

Recognizing the signs of peripheral artery disease and seeking prompt medical attention is crucial for preventing complications and preserving limb function and quality of life.

It is important to note that the risk and severity of these cardiovascular conditions can be influenced by a variety of factors, including family history, lifestyle habits, and the presence of other underlying health conditions. By understanding the common cardiovascular concerns faced by men over 50, you can take proactive steps to mitigate your risk and maintain a healthy heart.

Maintaining a Healthy Heart Through Diet and Exercise

One of the most powerful tools in your arsenal for preserving cardiovascular health is a comprehensive approach to diet and exercise. By adopting a healthy lifestyle, you can not only reduce your risk of developing cardiovascular problems but also actively manage and potentially reverse existing conditions.

1. Embracing a Heart-Healthy Diet
A well-balanced, nutrient-dense diet is essential for maintaining a healthy heart. When it comes to men's cardiovascular health, the following dietary considerations are particularly important:

- Increase intake of whole, unprocessed foods: Focus on incorporating a variety of fruits, vegetables, whole grains, lean proteins, and healthy fats into your meals.
  - Limit saturated and trans fats: Reduce the consumption of high-fat meats, full-fat dairy products, and processed foods, which can contribute to the buildup of harmful cholesterol.
  - Emphasize omega-3 fatty acids: Found in fatty fish, such as salmon, mackerel, and sardines, omega-3s can help lower triglyceride levels and reduce inflammation.
  - Manage sodium intake: Limit your consumption of high-sodium foods,

as excessive sodium can lead to or exacerbate hypertension.

- Stay hydrated: Drink plenty of water throughout the day to support overall cardiovascular function.

By making strategic dietary choices, you can actively support your heart health and reduce your risk of developing conditions like coronary artery disease, high blood pressure, and high cholesterol.

2. Incorporating Regular Physical Activity

Regular exercise is a cornerstone of cardiovascular health, and it becomes even more crucial as men age. Engaging in a well-rounded fitness routine can provide a multitude of benefits, including:

- Improving heart muscle function: Regular aerobic exercise, such as brisk walking, cycling, or swimming, can strengthen the heart and increase its efficiency in pumping blood.

- Lowering blood pressure: Physical activity can help reduce high blood pressure by improving blood vessel function and reducing vascular resistance.

- Enhancing cholesterol profiles: Exercise can help increase HDL (good) cholesterol levels while lowering LDL (bad) cholesterol and triglycerides.

- Maintaining a healthy weight: Regular physical activity, combined with a balanced diet, can help you achieve and maintain a healthy body weight, which is essential for cardiovascular health.

- Reducing the risk of diabetes: Exercise can improve insulin sensitivity and help prevent the development of type 2 diabetes, a major risk factor for heart disease.

Aim to incorporate a variety of exercise modalities into your routine, including aerobic activities, strength training, and flexibility exercises. This well-rounded approach can help you maintain cardiovascular fitness, improve overall physical function, and reduce your risk of age-related health problems.

3. Tailoring Your Fitness Plan

As men age, it's important to tailor your fitness plan to your individual needs, abilities, and any underlying health conditions you may have. Consult with your healthcare provider or a qualified exercise professional to develop a personalized exercise program that takes into account factors such as:

- Current cardiovascular health status: If you have a history of heart disease, high blood pressure, or other conditions, your exercise plan may need to be adapted to accommodate your specific needs.
- Mobility and flexibility: As you age, it's important to include exercises that maintain and improve your range of motion and flexibility, which can help prevent injuries and support overall cardiovascular health.
- Intensity and duration: Your exercise program should be designed to challenge you without overexerting your body. Start at a manageable intensity and gradually increase the duration and difficulty as your fitness improves.
- Recovery and rest: Adequate rest and recovery time are essential for allowing your body to adapt and repair itself, reducing the risk of injury and cardiovascular strain.

By collaborating with healthcare professionals and taking a personalized approach to your fitness routine, you can maximize the cardiovascular benefits of exercise while minimizing the risk of adverse events.

Managing Cardiovascular Risk Factors

In addition to a healthy diet and regular physical activity, effectively managing your cardiovascular risk factors is crucial for maintaining a strong and resilient heart. By addressing these modifiable risk factors, you can significantly reduce your chances of developing life-threatening cardiovascular conditions.

1. Blood Pressure Control
As mentioned earlier, hypertension is a significant risk factor for cardiovascular disease. Maintaining healthy blood pressure levels, typically defined

as less than 130/80 mmHg, is essential for preserving cardiovascular health.

This may involve a combination of lifestyle modifications, such as dietary changes, regular exercise, and stress management techniques, as well as the use of blood pressure-lowering medications if necessary. Consistent monitoring and close collaboration with your healthcare provider are key to effectively managing hypertension.

2. Cholesterol Management

High levels of LDL (bad) cholesterol and low levels of HDL (good) cholesterol can contribute to the development of atherosclerosis and increase the risk of heart disease. Regular cholesterol screenings and the implementation of a cholesterol-lowering strategy, which may include dietary changes, exercise, and potentially medication, can help optimize your cholesterol profile.

3. Diabetes and Metabolic Health

Type 2 diabetes is a major risk factor for cardiovascular disease, as it can lead to a host of related complications, such as high blood pressure, dyslipidemia, and inflammation. Maintaining tight control of your blood glucose levels through lifestyle modifications, medication management, and regular monitoring can significantly reduce your risk of developing diabetes-related cardiovascular problems.

4. Tobacco Cessation

Smoking is a well-established risk factor for a wide range of cardiovascular diseases, including heart attacks, strokes, and peripheral artery disease. Quitting smoking can have immediate and long-term benefits for your cardiovascular health, reducing your risk of these life-threatening conditions.

5. Stress Management

Chronic stress can have a detrimental impact on the cardiovascular system, contributing to the development of hypertension, inflammation, and other risk factors. Incorporating stress-reducing techniques, such as meditation, mindfulness practices, and regular relaxation activities, can help mitigate the negative effects of stress on your heart health.

6. Weight Management

Maintaining a healthy weight through a balanced diet and regular exercise can have a profound impact on your cardiovascular well-being. Excess weight, particularly around the abdomen, is associated with an increased risk of conditions like high blood pressure, high cholesterol, and type 2 diabetes, all of which can compromise heart health.

By proactively addressing and managing these key cardiovascular risk factors, you can take a significant step towards preserving your heart's health and longevity.

Navigating Cardiovascular Treatments and Interventions

In some cases, despite your best efforts to maintain a healthy lifestyle, you may still require medical intervention to manage cardiovascular conditions. Understanding the available treatment options and working closely with your healthcare team can help you make informed decisions and achieve the best possible outcomes.

1. Medication Management

Pharmacological interventions play a crucial role in the management of various cardiovascular conditions. Depending on your specific needs, your healthcare provider may prescribe medications to:

- Lower blood pressure
    - Improve cholesterol levels
    - Regulate heart rhythms
    - Reduce the risk of blood clots
    - Improve heart function in cases of heart failure

It is important to take these medications as prescribed, adhere to regular monitoring, and communicate any side effects or concerns to your healthcare provider.

2. Minimally Invasive Procedures

For certain cardiovascular conditions, such as coronary artery disease or valve issues, minimally invasive interventions may be recommended. These procedures, which often involve the use of catheters and small incisions, can help improve blood flow, restore proper heart function, and reduce the risk of more severe complications.

Examples of minimally invasive cardiovascular procedures include:
- Angioplasty and stent placement to open blocked arteries
- Transcatheter aortic valve replacement (TAVR) to treat aortic stenosis
- Catheter ablation to correct certain types of arrhythmias

3. Surgical Interventions

In more complex or advanced cases, traditional open-heart surgery may be necessary to address cardiovascular issues. These procedures, such as coronary artery bypass grafting, heart valve repairs or replacements, and surgical treatments for heart failure, are often reserved for situations where less invasive options are not suitable or have been exhausted.

While the prospect of undergoing surgery can be daunting, advancements in medical technology and surgical techniques have significantly improved the safety and outcomes of these interventions.

Regardless of the specific treatment approach, it is crucial to work closely with your healthcare team to understand the benefits, risks, and long-term implications of any cardiovascular intervention. Actively participating in the decision-making process and maintaining open communication can help you make informed choices and ensure the best possible outcome for your cardiovascular health.

Embracing a Proactive Approach to Heart Health

Maintaining a healthy cardiovascular system is not a one-time endeavor; it is a lifelong commitment that requires a proactive and comprehensive approach. By understanding the unique challenges faced by men over 50, embracing a heart-healthy lifestyle, and being willing to seek medical intervention when necessary, you can actively safeguard your heart and enjoy a vibrant, fulfilling life in the years to come.

Remember, the choices you make today have a profound impact on your cardiovascular well-being tomorrow. Embrace the power of preventive care, make mindful lifestyle choices, and remain vigilant in monitoring your heart health. With dedication and the right support, you can overcome the cardiovascular challenges of aging and thrive in the next chapter of your life.

Your heart is the cornerstone of your overall health and well-being. Treat it with the care and attention it deserves, and you will be rewarded with a strong, resilient cardiovascular system that can carry you through the adventures and joys of your later years.

CHAPTER 4

Maintaining Strong Musculoskeletal Health

As men transition into their later years, the gradual changes within the musculoskeletal system can have a profound impact on their overall health, mobility, and quality of life. From the gradual loss of bone density to the wear and tear on joints, the aging process presents a unique set of challenges that must be addressed proactively to ensure that you can maintain your independence, engage in physical activities, and continue to enjoy an active lifestyle.

In this chapter, we will delve into the key aspects of musculoskeletal health for men over 50. We'll explore the physiological changes that occur, the common conditions that may arise, and the essential strategies for preserving bone strength, muscle mass, and joint function through a comprehensive approach to exercise, nutrition, and targeted interventions.

Understanding the Aging Musculoskeletal System

The musculoskeletal system is a complex network of bones, joints, ligaments, tendons, and muscles that work together to provide structure, support, and mobility to the human body. As men age, this intricate system undergoes a gradual process of change and decline, which can have far-reaching consequences if not addressed proactively.

1. Bone Health Deterioration

One of the primary concerns associated with the aging musculoskeletal system is the gradual loss of bone density, a condition known as osteoporosis. As men grow older, the natural process of bone remodeling, where old bone is replaced by new bone, becomes less efficient, leading to a net loss of bone mass.

This decline in bone strength can increase the risk of fractures, particularly in the spine, hips, and wrists – areas that are prone to injury from falls or other impacts. Osteoporosis can have a significant impact on an individual's mobility, independence, and overall quality of life, making it a critical issue to address.

2. Muscle Mass Decline

Another hallmark of the aging musculoskeletal system is the gradual loss of muscle mass and strength, a condition known as sarcopenia. As men grow older, they experience a natural decline in the production of hormones, such as testosterone, which play a crucial role in maintaining muscle tissue.

This loss of muscle mass can lead to a reduction in strength, power, and physical function, making it more challenging to perform everyday tasks, engage in physical activities, and maintain independence. Sarcopenia can also increase the risk of falls and fractures, further compromising musculoskeletal health.

3. Joint Degeneration

The aging process also takes a toll on the joints, leading to the gradual degeneration of the cartilage that cushions the bones and facilitates smooth, pain-free movement. This condition, known as osteoarthritis, is one of the most common musculoskeletal disorders among older adults.

As the cartilage deteriorates, the bones can rub against each other, causing pain, inflammation, and a loss of range of motion. This can significantly impact an individual's ability to perform physical activities, leading to a more sedentary lifestyle and an increased risk of further musculoskeletal complications.

Understanding these age-related changes in the musculoskeletal system is the first step in developing an effective strategy for preserving bone strength, muscle mass, and joint function as you grow older.

Common Musculoskeletal Conditions in Men After 50

As men navigate the later stages of life, they face an increased risk of developing a variety of musculoskeletal conditions. It is crucial to be aware of these common issues and take proactive steps to manage them effectively.

1. Osteoporosis
   Osteoporosis, the gradual loss of bone density, is a significant concern for men over 50. This condition can lead to an increased risk of fractures, particularly in the spine, hips, and wrists, which can have a profound impact on mobility, independence, and quality of life.

Identifying and managing osteoporosis through a combination of lifestyle modifications, medication, and targeted interventions is essential for maintaining strong, healthy bones and reducing the risk of debilitating fractures.

2. Osteoarthritis
   Osteoarthritis, the gradual degeneration of the joint cartilage, is another common musculoskeletal condition that affects men as they age. This can lead to pain, stiffness, and a loss of range of motion in the affected joints, often the hips, knees, and hands.

Effective management of osteoarthritis may involve a combination of non-pharmacological interventions, such as weight management, exercise, and physical therapy, as well as the use of pain medications, joint injections, and potentially, surgical interventions in more severe cases.

3. Rotator Cuff Injuries

The shoulder, with its complex structure and range of motion, is particularly vulnerable to age-related injuries, such as rotator cuff tears. These injuries can cause pain, weakness, and a limited range of motion, often making it difficult to perform everyday tasks or engage in physical activities.

Addressing rotator cuff injuries may require a combination of conservative treatments, including physical therapy and anti-inflammatory medications, and in some cases, surgical interventions to repair or reconstruct the damaged tendons.

4. Lower Back Pain

Lower back pain is a common musculoskeletal complaint among older adults, often stemming from a variety of underlying causes, such as spinal degeneration, muscle imbalances, and joint dysfunction.

Effectively managing lower back pain may involve a multifaceted approach, including physical therapy, exercise, pain medication, and in some cases, interventional treatments like epidural injections or surgical procedures to address the underlying issues.

5. Foot and Ankle Conditions

As men age, they may also experience an increased incidence of foot and ankle conditions, such as plantar fasciitis, Achilles tendinitis, and ankle instability. These issues can significantly impact mobility, balance, and the ability to engage in physical activities.

Addressing foot and ankle problems may require a combination of appropriate footwear, physical therapy, custom orthotics, and in some cases, surgical interventions to correct structural abnormalities or repair damaged tissues.

It is important to note that the risk and severity of these musculoskeletal conditions can be influenced by a variety of factors, including lifestyle, injury history, underlying health conditions, and genetic predispositions. By understanding the common musculoskeletal concerns faced by men over 50, you can take proactive steps to mitigate your risk and maintain strong, healthy bones, muscles, and joints.

Preserving Bone Strength and Muscle Mass

Maintaining robust bone health and muscle mass is crucial for preserving overall musculoskeletal function, reducing the risk of injuries and fractures, and enabling an active, independent lifestyle as you grow older. By incorporating a comprehensive approach to bone and muscle health, you can take control of your musculoskeletal well-being.

1. Optimizing Bone Health

Maintaining strong, dense bones is essential for reducing the risk of osteoporosis and related fractures. Here are some key strategies for preserving bone strength:

a. Adequate Calcium and Vitamin D Intake

Calcium and vitamin D are essential nutrients for bone health. Aim to consume a diet rich in calcium-containing foods, such as dairy products, leafy greens, and fortified cereals. Additionally, ensure sufficient vitamin D intake, either through sun exposure, dietary sources, or supplements if necessary.

b. Weight-Bearing Exercise

Engaging in regular weight-bearing exercises, such as walking, jogging, or strength training, can help stimulate bone formation and improve bone density. These activities place a gentle stress on the bones, which helps to maintain their strength and resilience.

c. Targeted Bone-Building Supplements

In some cases, your healthcare provider may recommend the use of bone-building supplements, such as calcium, vitamin D, or bisphosphonate medications, to help preserve bone health and prevent the development of osteoporosis.

2. Maintaining Muscle Mass and Strength

Preserving muscle mass and strength is crucial for maintaining physical function, preventing falls and injuries, and supporting overall well-being. Incorporate the following strategies into your lifestyle:

a. Resistance Training

Engaging in regular resistance training exercises, such as weightlifting, bodyweight exercises, or resistance band workouts, can help stimulate muscle growth and maintain strength as you age.

b. Protein-Rich Diet

Ensuring adequate dietary protein intake is essential for supporting muscle health. Incorporate a variety of protein-rich foods, such as lean meats, poultry, fish, eggs, legumes, and dairy products, into your meals.

c. Optimizing Nutrition

In addition to protein, a well-balanced diet rich in fruits, vegetables, whole grains, and healthy fats can provide the necessary nutrients to support muscle growth and maintenance.

d. Hormonal Considerations

As men age, the gradual decline in testosterone production can contribute to the loss of muscle mass. Your healthcare provider may recommend strategies to address any hormonal imbalances, such as testosterone replacement therapy or other interventions.

3. Tailoring Your Musculoskeletal Fitness Plan

When designing your musculoskeletal fitness plan, it's essential to consider your individual needs, abilities, and any underlying health conditions you may have. Consult with a healthcare professional, such as an orthopedist, physical therapist, or exercise specialist, to develop a personalized program that addresses the following factors:

a. Current Musculoskeletal Health Status

If you have a history of musculoskeletal injuries, conditions like osteoporosis or osteoarthritis, or any other underlying issues, your fitness plan should be tailored to accommodate your specific needs and limitations.

b. Mobility and Flexibility

As you age, it's crucial to include exercises that maintain and improve your range of motion, flexibility, and balance. This can help prevent injuries and support overall musculoskeletal function.

c. Intensity and Progression

Your exercise program should be designed to challenge you appropriately, starting at a manageable intensity and gradually increasing the difficulty over time as your fitness improves.

d. Recovery and Rest

Adequate rest and recovery time are essential for allowing your muscles and bones to adapt and repair themselves. Incorporating rest days and allowing for proper recovery between sessions is key to avoiding overuse injuries and supporting long-term musculoskeletal health.

By taking a comprehensive, personalized approach to preserving bone strength and muscle mass, you can proactively address the musculoskeletal challenges associated with aging and maintain your physical independence and quality of life.

Preventing and Managing Joint Issues

Joint health is a critical component of overall musculoskeletal well-being, and addressing joint-related concerns is essential for maintaining mobility, reducing pain, and enabling an active lifestyle as you grow older.

1. Osteoarthritis Management

As mentioned earlier, osteoarthritis is a common joint condition that affects many men over 50. Effective management of osteoarthritis may involve a combination of the following strategies:

a. Weight Management

Maintaining a healthy body weight can significantly reduce the stress and strain on weight-bearing joints, such as the hips and knees, and help slow the progression of osteoarthritis.

b. Exercise and Physical Therapy

Engaging in low-impact exercises, such as swimming, cycling, or gentle resistance training, can help strengthen the muscles around the affected joints, improve range of motion, and reduce pain. Working with a physical therapist can also help develop an effective, personalized exercise plan.

c. Pain Management

Over-the-counter or prescription pain medications, as well as topical creams or ointments, can help alleviate joint pain and inflammation associated with osteoarthritis. In some cases, corticosteroid injections may be recommended to provide temporary relief.

d. Surgical Interventions

For more severe cases of osteoarthritis, when conservative treatments have been exhausted, joint replacement surgery, such as total hip or knee replacement, may be considered to restore function and reduce pain.

2. Injury Prevention and Rehabilitation

Preventing joint injuries and effectively rehabilitating any existing issues is crucial for maintaining long-term joint health and reducing the risk of further complications.

a. Proper Warm-Up and Cool-Down

Incorporating a thorough warm-up and cool-down routine into your exercise regimen can help prepare your joints for physical activity and reduce the risk of acute injuries.

b. Supportive Equipment and Bracing

Using appropriate protective equipment, such as joint braces or supports, can help stabilize and support vulnerable joints during physical activity, reducing the risk of injury.

c. Physical Therapy and Rehabilitation

If you do experience a joint injury, working with a physical therapist to develop a comprehensive rehabilitation plan can help restore function, improve range of motion, and prevent the development of chronic issues.

3. Promoting Joint Health Through Nutrition

Certain dietary choices can also play a role in supporting joint health and reducing the risk of joint-related issues.

a. Anti-Inflammatory Foods

Incorporating foods rich in omega-3 fatty acids, such as fatty fish, walnuts, and flaxseeds, as well as antioxidant-rich fruits and vegetables, can help reduce inflammation and support joint function.

b. Collagen and Glucosamine Supplements

Some research suggests that supplements containing collagen or glucosamine may provide some benefits for joint health, although the evidence is mixed. Consult with your healthcare provider before starting any new supplement regimen.

c. Hydration and Joint Lubrication

Ensuring adequate hydration by drinking plenty of water can help maintain the lubricating properties of the synovial fluid that cushions the joints, promoting smooth and pain-free movement.

By taking a multifaceted approach to joint health, you can proactively address the challenges of aging and maintain your mobility, independence, and quality of life well into your later years.

Embracing a Holistic Approach to Musculoskeletal Health

Preserving strong, healthy bones, muscles, and joints requires a comprehensive and holistic approach that addresses the various aspects of your musculoskeletal well-being. By incorporating the following key elements into your lifestyle, you can take control of your musculoskeletal health and set the stage for a fulfilling, active future.

1. Regular Check-ups and Monitoring

Consistent communication with your healthcare providers, including your primary care physician, orthopedist, or physical therapist, is essential for monitoring the health of your musculoskeletal system. Regular check-ups, screenings, and assessments can help identify any underlying issues or risk factors before they escalate.

2. Proactive Lifestyle Modifications

Adopting a lifestyle that prioritizes musculoskeletal health is crucial for maintaining strength, mobility, and function as you age. This includes regular exercise, a balanced and nutrient-rich diet, and the incorporation of targeted interventions, such as strength training, flexibility exercises, and fall prevention strategies.

3. Injury Prevention and Rehabilitation

Being proactive in preventing musculoskeletal injuries and effectively rehabilitating any existing issues is key to preserving long-term joint and muscle health. Incorporating proper warm-up and cool-down routines, using supportive equipment, and working with physical therapists can help minimize the risk of injuries and facilitate a successful recovery.

4. Collaboration with Healthcare Providers

When it comes to managing musculoskeletal health, it's important to work closely with your healthcare team, including your primary care physician, orthopedists, physical therapists, and any other relevant specialists. This collaborative approach can help ensure that your specific needs are addressed, and the most appropriate treatments and interventions are implemented.

5. Emotional Well-Being and Resilience

The musculoskeletal system is not just a physical construct; it is also closely linked to our emotional and psychological well-being. Factors like stress, anxiety, and depression can have a negative impact on musculoskeletal health, contributing to issues such as chronic pain, decreased mobility, and reduced exercise motivation.

By prioritizing your emotional well-being, through practices like stress management, mindfulness, and social engagement, you can foster a greater sense of resilience and support the overall health of your musculoskeletal system.

Embracing the Journey of Lifelong Musculoskeletal Health

As you navigate the journey of aging, it's essential to approach your musculoskeletal health with a proactive, holistic, and long-term perspective. By understanding the unique challenges you may face, adopting proven strategies for maintaining bone strength, muscle mass, and joint function, and collaborating closely with your healthcare providers, you can take control of your musculoskeletal well-being and set the stage for a vibrant, active, and independent future.

Remember, the choices you make today have a profound impact on your physical capabilities, mobility, and overall quality of life in the years to come. Embrace the power of prevention, commit to a lifestyle that prioritizes musculoskeletal health, and trust that your efforts will be rewarded with the ability to continue pursuing the activities, adventures, and experiences that bring you joy and fulfillment.

Your musculoskeletal system is the foundation upon which your physical independence and vitality rest. Treat it with the care and attention it deserves, and you will be well on your way to maintaining a strong, resilient, and healthy body that can carry you through the decades ahead.

CHAPTER 5

Addressing Hormonal Changes

As men transition into the second half of their lives, one of the most significant physiological changes they experience is a gradual decline in hormone production, particularly testosterone. This hormonal shift can have far-reaching consequences, affecting everything from sexual function and body composition to mood, energy levels, and overall well-being.

In this chapter, we will delve into the complex world of male hormonal changes, exploring the implications of declining testosterone and the strategies for effectively addressing this critical aspect of aging. We'll discuss the importance of understanding your hormone levels, the potential benefits and risks of hormone replacement therapy, and the role of lifestyle modifications in maintaining hormonal balance.

Understanding the Testosterone Decline

Testosterone, the primary male sex hormone, plays a crucial role in a man's physical, sexual, and emotional well-being. However, as men age, their testosterone levels gradually decline, a process known as andropause or late-onset hypogonadism.

1. The Natural Decline of Testosterone

Starting around the age of 30, men typically experience a gradual, yet steady, reduction in their testosterone production, with levels decreasing by approximately 1% per year. By the time a man reaches his 50s or 60s, his testosterone levels may be significantly lower than they were in his younger years.

This age-related decline in testosterone can have a profound impact on various aspects of a man's health and quality of life, including:

- Sexual function and libido
    - Muscle mass and strength
    - Bone density
    - Energy levels and fatigue
    - Mood and cognitive function
    - Body composition and weight management

Understanding the natural progression of testosterone decline is crucial for recognizing when intervention may be necessary and for developing an effective strategy to manage the associated changes.

2. Diagnosing Testosterone Deficiency

Determining whether a man is experiencing a clinically significant testosterone deficiency, known as hypogonadism, requires a comprehensive evaluation by a healthcare provider. This typically involves a thorough medical history, physical examination, and a series of blood tests to measure the individual's testosterone levels.

It's important to note that a single low testosterone reading does not necessarily indicate a problem; testosterone levels can fluctuate throughout the day and can be influenced by a variety of factors, such as stress, illness, and even the time of day when the blood sample was taken.

To accurately diagnose hypogonadism, healthcare providers often look for a pattern of consistently low testosterone levels, accompanied by the presence of specific symptoms and the exclusion of other underlying health conditions that could be contributing to the hormonal imbalance.

3. Symptoms of Testosterone Deficiency

The symptoms associated with testosterone deficiency can vary widely from individual to individual, but some of the most common include:

- Decreased libido and sexual function
    - Erectile dysfunction
    - Reduced muscle mass and strength
    - Increased body fat, particularly around the abdomen
    - Fatigue and decreased energy levels
    - Mood changes, such as irritability, depression, or decreased motivation
    - Decreased bone density and increased risk of osteoporosis
    - Impaired cognitive function, including memory and concentration issues

By being aware of these potential symptoms, men can be proactive in seeking medical attention and addressing any underlying hormonal imbalances.

Exploring Hormone Replacement Therapy Options

One of the primary interventions for addressing testosterone deficiency is hormone replacement therapy (HRT). This approach involves the administration of exogenous testosterone, either through injections, transdermal gels or patches, or oral medications, to restore the body's testosterone levels to a more youthful range.

1. Benefits of Testosterone Replacement Therapy

When used appropriately and under the guidance of a healthcare provider, testosterone replacement therapy can provide a variety of benefits for men experiencing hypogonadism, including:

- Improved sexual function and libido
    - Increased muscle mass and strength
    - Enhanced bone density and reduced fracture risk
    - Improved energy levels and reduced fatigue
    - Better mood and cognitive function
    - Potential reduction in the risk of certain chronic conditions, such as cardiovascular disease and type 2 diabetes

By addressing the underlying hormonal imbalance, testosterone replacement therapy can help restore a man's physical, sexual, and emotional well-being, significantly enhancing his quality of life.

2. Potential Risks and Considerations

While testosterone replacement therapy can be highly beneficial, it is essential to be aware of the potential risks and carefully weigh the pros and cons with your healthcare provider. Some of the potential risks and side effects associated with testosterone therapy include:

- Prostate enlargement and increased risk of prostate cancer
    - Elevated red blood cell count, which can increase the risk of blood clots
    - Sleep apnea or worsening of existing sleep apnea
    - Fluid retention and edema
    - Acne or oily skin
    - Decreased testicular size and sperm production

Additionally, it's important to note that the long-term safety and efficacy of testosterone replacement therapy, particularly for older men, are still being actively researched. Your healthcare provider will carefully evaluate your individual circumstances and health history to determine the appropriate course of action.

3. Personalized Approach to Testosterone Therapy

When it comes to testosterone replacement therapy, a one-size-fits-all approach is not effective. Each individual's needs and response to treatment can vary significantly, necessitating a personalized approach.

Your healthcare provider will work with you to determine the appropriate dosage, delivery method, and monitoring protocols to ensure that your testosterone levels are restored to a healthy range without causing any adverse effects. Regular follow-up appointments, blood tests, and ongoing assessment are crucial for optimizing the benefits and minimizing the risks of testosterone therapy.

Embracing Lifestyle Modifications for Hormonal Balance

While hormone replacement therapy can be a valuable tool in addressing testosterone deficiency, it is not the only approach. Incorporating lifestyle modifications can also play a crucial role in supporting hormonal balance and overall well-being as men age.

1. Maintaining a Healthy Weight

Excess body weight, particularly around the midsection, can have a negative impact on testosterone levels. Carrying extra weight, especially in the form of abdominal fat, is associated with increased aromatization – the conversion of testosterone to estrogen – which can further exacerbate hormonal imbalances.

By achieving and maintaining a healthy body weight through a balanced diet and regular physical activity, men can help support their natural testosterone production and reduce the risk of associated health problems.

2. Regular Exercise and Physical Activity

Engaging in regular exercise, both aerobic and resistance training, can be a powerful tool for supporting hormonal balance. Cardiovascular workouts, such as brisk walking, cycling, or swimming, have been shown to help increase testosterone levels, while strength training can help preserve and even build muscle mass, which is closely linked to healthy testosterone production.

It's important to find an exercise routine that you enjoy and can stick to consistently, as the benefits of physical activity on hormone levels are cumulative and can compound over time.

3. Stress Management and Relaxation

Chronic stress can have a significant impact on the body's hormone production, including the release of cortisol, which can interfere with the synthesis and utilization of testosterone. Incorporating stress management techniques, such as meditation, deep breathing exercises, or yoga, can help mitigate the negative effects of stress on hormonal balance.

Additionally, ensuring that you get adequate sleep and engage in relaxation activities can further support your body's natural hormone regulation processes.

4. Dietary Considerations

The foods you consume can also play a role in supporting hormonal balance. Incorporating a nutrient-dense, whole-food-based diet rich in healthy fats, proteins, and complex carbohydrates can provide the building blocks for optimal testosterone production.

Some specific dietary recommendations include:
- Consuming healthy fats, such as those found in nuts, seeds, avocados, and fatty fish
- Eating adequate amounts of high-quality protein from sources like lean meats, eggs, and legumes
- Limiting processed foods, refined carbohydrates, and added sugars, which can disrupt hormonal balance

Additionally, certain supplements, such as vitamin D, zinc, and ashwagandha, have been shown to have a positive impact on testosterone levels in some individuals, although the research is still ongoing. Always consult with your healthcare provider before starting any supplement regimen.

5. Maintaining a Positive Mindset

The connection between the mind and the body's hormonal system is well-established. Cultivating a positive, resilient mindset and engaging in practices that support emotional well-being can have a beneficial effect on hormone production and overall health.

Techniques such as mindfulness, cognitive-behavioral therapy, and social engagement can help manage stress, improve mood, and foster a sense of purpose – all of which can contribute to a more favorable hormonal profile.

Integrating Hormone Management into Your Holistic Health Plan

Addressing hormonal changes, particularly the decline in testosterone, is a critical component of a comprehensive men's health strategy. By taking a multifaceted approach that combines medical interventions, lifestyle modifications, and a focus on overall well-being, you can effectively manage the hormonal shifts associated with aging and maintain optimal physical, sexual, and emotional functioning.

1. Collaborate with Healthcare Professionals

Developing a strong partnership with your healthcare providers, including your primary care physician, endocrinologist, or urologist, is essential for managing hormonal changes. These professionals can help you navigate the complex landscape of hormone replacement therapy, interpret your test results, and customize a treatment plan that aligns with your individual needs and preferences.

Regular check-ups, open communication, and a collaborative decision-making process will ensure that your hormonal health is continuously monitored and that any necessary adjustments to your treatment plan are made in a timely manner.

2. Prioritize Preventive Measures

While hormone replacement therapy may be necessary in some cases, it's important to also focus on preventive strategies that can help maintain hormonal balance and overall well-being. This includes adopting a healthy lifestyle, managing stress, and engaging in regular physical activity – all of which can help support the body's natural hormone production and regulation.

By taking a proactive approach, you can potentially delay or even prevent the onset of significant hormonal imbalances, reducing the need for more intensive interventions down the line.

3. Embrace a Holistic Perspective

Hormonal changes do not exist in isolation; they are intrinsically linked to various other aspects of your health and well-being. By adopting a holistic perspective, you can ensure that your hormonal management strategy is integrated into a comprehensive plan that addresses your physical, mental, and emotional needs.

This may involve addressing other age-related health concerns, such as cardiovascular health, cognitive function, or musculoskeletal strength, and ensuring that your hormonal management plan is aligned with and supportive of your overall wellness goals.

4. Monitor and Adjust as Needed

Hormonal balance is not a static state; it is a dynamic process that can fluctuate over time. Regularly monitoring your hormone levels, paying attention to any changes in your symptoms, and working closely with your healthcare providers to make necessary adjustments to your treatment plan are essential for maintaining optimal hormonal health.

By embracing a continuous improvement mindset and remaining adaptable, you can navigate the ebb and flow of hormonal changes with confidence and ensure that your management strategy evolves along with your needs.

Embracing the Journey of Hormonal Wellness

As men navigate the later stages of life, the changes in their hormonal landscape can be both challenging and transformative. By understanding the natural decline in testosterone, exploring the benefits and considerations of hormone replacement therapy, and incorporating lifestyle modifications to support hormonal balance, you can take an active role in managing this critical aspect of your well-being.

Remember, your hormonal health is not just about sexual function or body composition; it is a crucial component of your overall physical, mental, and emotional well-being. By addressing hormonal changes proactively and integrating this aspect of your health into a holistic wellness plan, you can unlock a renewed sense of vitality, resilience, and fulfillment in the years to come.

Embrace the journey of hormonal wellness, collaborate with your healthcare team, and trust that the steps you take today will pave the way for a vibrant, empowered, and rewarding second half of life.

CHAPTER 6

I mproving Cognitive Function

As men enter the later stages of life, one of the most significant health concerns that often arises is the potential decline in cognitive function. The aging process can bring about subtle changes in memory, problem-solving abilities, and overall mental acuity, which can have a profound impact on an individual's independence, quality of life, and sense of self.

However, the news is not all grim. While cognitive decline is a natural part of the aging process, it is not an inevitable outcome. By understanding the underlying causes, adopting proactive lifestyle strategies, and incorporating targeted interventions, men over 50 can take control of their brain health and preserve their cognitive capabilities well into their later years.

In this chapter, we will explore the complexities of age-related cognitive changes, delve into the factors that can influence mental function, and provide a comprehensive plan for enhancing memory, sharpening mental acuity, and preventing or delaying the onset of more severe cognitive impairments.

Understanding Age-Related Cognitive Changes

The human brain is a remarkably complex and dynamic organ, and as we grow older, it undergoes a gradual transformation that can impact various aspects of cognitive function. It's important to understand the nuances of these age-related changes to better address and manage them.

1. Normal Age-Related Cognitive Decline

As men transition into their 50s, 60s, and beyond, they may begin to experience subtle changes in their cognitive abilities, such as:

- Slower processing speed: The brain's ability to quickly process and respond to information may gradually decline.
- Reduced working memory: The temporary storage and manipulation of information necessary for tasks like problem-solving may become more challenging.
- Difficulty with new learning: Acquiring and retaining new information or skills may require more effort and repetition.
- Occasionally misplacing items or forgetting names: Minor memory lapses may become more common.

These changes are a natural part of the aging process and do not necessarily indicate the presence of a more serious cognitive disorder. They are often subtle and may not significantly interfere with an individual's daily functioning or independence.

2. Mild Cognitive Impairment

In some cases, the cognitive changes experienced with aging may be more pronounced, leading to a condition known as mild cognitive impairment (MCI). MCI is characterized by a noticeable decline in cognitive abilities that is greater than what would be expected for a person's age, but not severe enough to interfere significantly with daily activities.

Individuals with MCI may experience more pronounced memory issues, difficulty with problem-solving, or challenges in maintaining focus and attention. While MCI does not necessarily lead to dementia, it can increase the risk of developing more severe cognitive disorders, such as Alzheimer's disease, over time.

3. Dementia and Alzheimer's Disease

At the more severe end of the spectrum, some men may develop age-related cognitive disorders, such as Alzheimer's disease or other forms of dementia. These conditions involve the progressive deterioration of cognitive functions, including memory, language, problem-solving, and decision-making abilities, to the point where they significantly interfere with an individual's daily life and independence.

While the development of these more serious cognitive impairments is not an inevitable outcome of aging, it is important to be aware of the risk factors and to seek prompt medical attention if concerning symptoms arise.

Understanding the Factors that Influence Cognitive Function

Cognitive function is the result of a complex interplay between various biological, lifestyle, and environmental factors. By identifying and addressing the key determinants of brain health, men over 50 can take proactive steps to maintain and even enhance their mental capabilities.

1. Biological Factors

The aging process brings about physiological changes within the brain that can impact cognitive function. These include:

- Decreased brain volume and connectivity: As we grow older, the brain may experience a gradual reduction in size and a decline in the connections between different regions, which can impair overall cognitive performance.
- Inflammation and oxidative stress: Chronic inflammation and the accumulation of oxidative damage can contribute to age-related cognitive decline.
- Vascular health: Poor cardiovascular health, such as high blood pressure or atherosclerosis, can compromise the brain's blood supply and oxygen delivery, leading to cognitive impairments.
- Hormonal changes: The gradual decline in hormones, such as testosterone

and thyroid hormones, can also have an impact on cognitive function.

2. Lifestyle Factors

The choices we make in our day-to-day lives can have a profound influence on our cognitive health. Key lifestyle factors include:

- Physical activity: Regular exercise has been shown to improve brain function, enhance neuroplasticity (the brain's ability to adapt and change), and potentially delay the onset of cognitive decline.
- Diet and nutrition: A balanced, nutrient-rich diet, including foods rich in antioxidants, healthy fats, and essential vitamins and minerals, can support optimal brain health.
- Sleep and stress management: Adequate, high-quality sleep and effective stress-reduction techniques can help maintain cognitive function and prevent the negative effects of chronic stress on the brain.
- Intellectual stimulation and social engagement: Challenging the brain through learning, problem-solving, and social interaction can help build cognitive reserves and promote mental resilience.

3. Environmental Factors

The environment in which we live and work can also impact cognitive function. Exposure to certain toxins, pollutants, or traumatic brain injuries can potentially contribute to cognitive decline over time.

Additionally, factors such as education level, socioeconomic status, and access to healthcare can influence an individual's cognitive health and risk of developing age-related cognitive disorders.

By understanding the multifaceted factors that shape cognitive function, men over 50 can take a proactive and comprehensive approach to preserving and enhancing their mental capabilities.

Enhancing Memory and Mental Acuity

One of the primary goals in addressing age-related cognitive changes is to maintain and even improve memory, problem-solving abilities, and overall mental sharpness. By incorporating a combination of lifestyle modifications, cognitive training, and targeted interventions, men can take control of their brain health and unlock their full cognitive potential.

1. Adopting a Brain-Healthy Lifestyle

Implementing a comprehensive lifestyle plan that prioritizes brain health is a foundational step in preserving and enhancing cognitive function. This includes:

a. Regular Physical Activity

Engaging in regular physical exercise, such as aerobic activities, strength training, and balance exercises, can help improve blood flow to the brain, promote the growth of new brain cells, and enhance neuroplasticity.

b. Balanced, Nutrient-Dense Diet

Consuming a diet rich in antioxidants, healthy fats, complex carbohydrates, and essential vitamins and minerals can provide the necessary fuel for optimal brain function. Foods like leafy greens, fatty fish, berries, and nuts are particularly beneficial for cognitive health.

c. Sufficient, High-Quality Sleep

Ensuring adequate, restorative sleep is crucial for memory consolidation, cognitive processing, and overall brain health. Establishing a consistent sleep routine and practicing good sleep hygiene can help support cognitive function.

d. Stress Management and Relaxation

Chronic stress can have a detrimental impact on the brain, impairing memory, concentration, and problem-solving abilities. Incorporating stress-reduction techniques, such as meditation, mindfulness, or relaxation exercises, can help mitigate the negative effects of stress on cognitive function.

2. Engaging in Cognitive Training and Brain Exercises

Challenging the brain through various cognitive training activities and brain exercises can help maintain and even enhance mental acuity as men age. Some effective strategies include:

a. Puzzles and Brain Teasers

Engaging in puzzles, crosswords, sudoku, and other mentally stimulating activities can help improve problem-solving skills, boost memory, and promote overall cognitive flexibility.

b. Learning New Skills

Acquiring new skills, such as learning a new language, playing a musical instrument, or coding, can help activate different regions of the brain and promote the development of new neural pathways.

c. Memory-Enhancing Techniques

Practicing memory-enhancing techniques, such as mnemonics, visualization, or memory palace strategies, can help strengthen memory recall and retention.

d. Computer-Based Cognitive Training Programs

Specialized cognitive training programs, delivered through computer or mobile applications, can provide a structured and personalized approach to improving various cognitive domains, such as attention, processing speed, and working memory.

3. Incorporating Targeted Interventions

In some cases, targeted interventions or therapies may be recommended to address specific cognitive challenges or to support overall brain health. These may include:

a. Cognitive Rehabilitation Therapy

Cognitive rehabilitation therapy, provided by trained healthcare professionals, can help individuals develop strategies and compensatory techniques to address specific cognitive deficits, such as memory impairments or executive function challenges.

b. Neurofeedback Training

Neurofeedback is a type of biofeedback that uses real-time monitoring of brain activity to help individuals learn to self-regulate their brain function, potentially leading to improvements in cognitive performance.

c. Prescription Medications

In certain cases, healthcare providers may prescribe medications, such as cholinesterase inhibitors or memantine, to help manage the symptoms of mild cognitive impairment or dementia. It's important to consult with your healthcare provider to discuss the potential risks and benefits of these interventions.

4. Addressing Underlying Health Conditions

Certain underlying health conditions, such as cardiovascular disease, diabetes, or thyroid imbalances, can have a direct impact on cognitive function. By addressing and managing these underlying issues, men can potentially mitigate the negative effects on their brain health.

Collaborating with healthcare professionals, such as primary care physicians, neurologists, or geriatric specialists, is crucial for identifying and effectively managing any underlying conditions that may be contributing to cognitive decline.

Preventing and Managing Age-Related Cognitive Decline

While the aging process inevitably brings about some changes in cognitive function, the good news is that men over 50 can take proactive steps to prevent or delay the onset of more severe cognitive impairments. By adopting a comprehensive approach that addresses the various factors influencing brain health, individuals can maintain their independence, enhance their quality of life, and continue to thrive in their later years.

1. Promoting Cognitive Reserve

The concept of cognitive reserve refers to the brain's ability to adapt and compensate for age-related changes or damage, allowing individuals to maintain cognitive function despite the presence of underlying neuropathology. By engaging in activities that build cognitive reserve, men can potentially delay or mitigate the effects of age-related cognitive decline.

Strategies for promoting cognitive reserve include:
- Pursuing lifelong learning and intellectual stimulation
- Engaging in physically, socially, and mentally active lifestyles
- Maintaining a healthy, balanced diet and regular exercise regimen
- Addressing and managing any underlying health conditions

2. Early Detection and Intervention

Regularly monitoring cognitive function and seeking prompt medical attention for any concerning changes or symptoms is crucial for effective management of age-related cognitive disorders. Early detection and intervention can make a significant difference in the trajectory of cognitive decline and the ability to maintain independence and quality of life.

This may involve:
- Routine cognitive assessments and screenings with healthcare providers
- Seeking evaluation and diagnosis for any suspected cognitive impairments
- Collaborating with healthcare professionals to develop a personalized management plan

3. Caregiver Support and Education

As men grow older, it's important to involve their loved ones and caregivers in the process of maintaining and supporting cognitive health. Educating family members and caregivers about age-related cognitive changes, the early signs of cognitive decline, and effective strategies for providing support can help ensure a comprehensive approach to brain health.

Additionally, connecting with support groups or community resources can provide valuable information, emotional support, and practical guidance for both individuals experiencing cognitive challenges and their loved ones.

4. Maintaining a Positive Outlook and Purpose

Cultivating a positive mindset and a sense of purpose can play a crucial role in preserving cognitive function and overall well-being as men age. Engaging in activities that bring joy, meaning, and a sense of accomplishment can help maintain cognitive stimulation, foster social connections, and promote a resilient, adaptive mindset.

By embracing a proactive, multifaceted approach to cognitive health, men over 50 can take control of their brain function, maintain their independence, and continue to thrive in their later years.

Embracing the Journey of Cognitive Wellness

As men navigate the complexities of aging, preserving cognitive function and mental acuity should be a top priority. By understanding the nuances of age-related cognitive changes, addressing the various factors that influence brain health, and incorporating a comprehensive plan for enhancing memory and mental sharpness, individuals can take an active role in safeguarding their cognitive well-being.

Remember, cognitive decline is not an inevitable outcome of aging. With the right mindset, targeted interventions, and a commitment to lifelong learning and brain-healthy habits, men can unlock their full cognitive potential and continue to engage in the activities, pursuits, and relationships that bring them joy and fulfillment.

Embrace the journey of cognitive wellness, collaborate with healthcare professionals, and trust that the steps you take today will pave the way for a future filled with mental clarity, resilience, and the ability to navigate the world with confidence and purpose.

CHAPTER 7

Mastering Sleep and Stress Management

As men transition into their 50s, 60s, and beyond, the importance of maintaining a healthy sleep-wake cycle and effectively managing stress becomes increasingly crucial. These two interrelated aspects of well-being can have a profound impact on an individual's physical, mental, and emotional health, with far-reaching consequences for overall quality of life.

In this chapter, we will delve into the critical role of sleep and stress management in the lives of men over 50. We'll explore the physiological changes that can affect sleep patterns and the body's response to stress, and we'll provide a comprehensive plan for optimizing sleep quality, implementing effective stress-reduction techniques, and maintaining a balanced, resilient approach to the challenges of aging.

The Importance of Quality Sleep

Sleep is a fundamental biological necessity, playing a crucial role in physical restoration, cognitive function, and emotional well-being. As men grow older, however, the sleep-wake cycle can become disrupted, leading to a host of problems that can significantly impact their overall health and quality of life.

1. Age-Related Changes in Sleep Patterns

The aging process brings about various physiological changes that can affect sleep quality and duration. Some of the common sleep-related challenges faced by men over 50 include:

a. Reduced sleep efficiency: Older adults often experience a decline in the amount of time they spend in deep, restorative sleep stages, leading to more fragmented and less restful sleep.

b. Increased sleep fragmentation: Older men may experience more frequent awakenings throughout the night, disrupting the continuity of their sleep.

c. Earlier bedtimes and wake times: As men age, their circadian rhythms (the body's internal clock) can shift, causing them to feel sleepy earlier in the evening and wake up earlier in the morning.

d. Increased prevalence of sleep disorders: Conditions like sleep apnea, restless leg syndrome, and insomnia become more common with age, further compromising sleep quality.

Understanding these age-related changes in sleep patterns is the first step in developing an effective strategy for optimizing sleep and preventing the negative consequences of poor sleep.

2. The Impact of Poor Sleep on Health

Inadequate or poor-quality sleep can have a profound impact on an individual's physical, mental, and emotional well-being. Some of the potential consequences of poor sleep in men over 50 include:

a. Increased risk of chronic diseases: Insufficient sleep has been linked to an elevated risk of conditions like cardiovascular disease, diabetes, and certain types of cancer.

b. Cognitive impairments: Sleep deprivation can negatively affect memory, concentration, decision-making, and overall cognitive function.

c. Mood disturbances: Lack of sleep can contribute to the development or exacerbation of mental health issues, such as depression and anxiety.

d. Reduced physical function and increased risk of falls: Poor sleep can impair balance, coordination, and muscle function, increasing the likelihood of falls and injuries.

e. Decreased quality of life and overall well-being: Chronic sleep disturbances can significantly diminish an individual's overall quality of life, leading to a reduced sense of vitality and enjoyment.

Recognizing the profound impact of sleep on various aspects of health is essential for men over 50 to prioritize the optimization of their sleep-wake patterns.

Implementing Effective Sleep Strategies

Improving sleep quality and duration is a crucial aspect of maintaining overall health and well-being as men age. By incorporating a comprehensive approach to sleep optimization, individuals can reap the numerous benefits of restful, restorative sleep.

1. Establishing a Consistent Sleep Routine

One of the foundational strategies for improving sleep is the development of a consistent sleep routine. This involves:

a. Maintaining a regular sleep-wake schedule: Going to bed and waking up at the same time, even on weekends, can help regulate the body's internal clock and promote better sleep quality.

b. Creating a sleep-conducive environment: Ensuring that the bedroom is dark, cool, and quiet can help create an optimal environment for restful sleep.

c. Implementing a pre-bedtime routine: Engaging in relaxing activities, such as reading, light stretching, or meditation, can help signal to the body that it's time to wind down and prepare for sleep.

2. Addressing Sleep Disorders

If an individual is experiencing persistent sleep disturbances, it's important to seek medical attention to identify and address any underlying sleep disorders, such as sleep apnea, restless leg syndrome, or insomnia. Treatments may include:

a. Continuous positive airway pressure (CPAP) therapy for sleep apnea

b. Medications or cognitive-behavioral therapy for insomnia

c. Lifestyle modifications and supplements for restless leg syndrome

Collaborating with healthcare providers, such as sleep specialists or primary care physicians, is crucial for developing an effective treatment plan.

3. Incorporating Sleep-Promoting Habits

In addition to establishing a consistent sleep routine and addressing any sleep disorders, men over 50 can incorporate various sleep-promoting habits into their daily lives, such as:

a. Limiting screen time before bed: The blue light emitted by electronic devices can disrupt the body's natural sleep-wake cycle.

b. Avoiding caffeine, nicotine, and alcohol close to bedtime: These substances can interfere with sleep quality and duration.

c. Engaging in regular physical activity: Exercise can help improve sleep, but it's important to avoid vigorous workouts close to bedtime.

d. Practicing relaxation techniques: Mindfulness, deep breathing, or progressive muscle relaxation can help calm the mind and body, facilitating better sleep.

4. Monitoring and Tracking Sleep

Regularly monitoring and tracking sleep patterns can provide valuable insights into an individual's sleep quality and help identify any potential issues. This can be done through a variety of methods, including:

a. Sleep tracking apps or wearable devices
　　b. Sleep journals or logs
　　c. Discussions with healthcare providers during routine check-ups

By closely monitoring sleep patterns, men over 50 can make informed decisions about adjusting their sleep habits and seeking professional help when necessary.

Mastering Stress Management

Stress is a ubiquitous part of the human experience, and as men transition into their later years, they may face a unique set of stressors that can have a profound impact on their physical and mental well-being. Developing effective strategies for stress management is crucial for maintaining a high quality of life and promoting overall health.

1. Understanding the Physiological Response to Stress
　　When the body is under stress, it activates the sympathetic nervous system, triggering a cascade of physiological changes, including the release of hormones like cortisol. This stress response is designed to help the body cope with immediate threats, but chronic, unmanaged stress can have detrimental effects on various body systems, including:

a. Cardiovascular health: Chronic stress can contribute to the development of hypertension, heart disease, and other cardiovascular problems.
　　b. Metabolic health: Stress can disrupt glucose regulation and lead to weight gain, insulin resistance, and an increased risk of type 2 diabetes.
　　c. Immune function: Prolonged stress can weaken the immune system, making individuals more susceptible to illness and infection.
　　d. Cognitive function: Chronic stress can impair memory, concentration, and decision-making abilities.
　　e. Mental health: Stress is a major risk factor for the development of conditions like depression, anxiety, and burnout.

Understanding the physiological mechanisms underlying the stress response is the first step in developing effective strategies for stress management.

2. Identifying Sources of Stress

The first step in managing stress is to identify the specific sources or triggers that are contributing to an individual's stress levels. Common sources of stress for men over 50 may include:

a. Retirement and financial concerns

b. Health issues or the care of aging parents

c. Relationship challenges or the loss of a loved one

d. Feelings of isolation or lack of social connection

e. Uncertainty or anxiety about the future

By recognizing the specific stressors in their lives, men can tailor their stress management strategies to address the underlying issues more effectively.

3. Implementing Stress-Reduction Techniques

Once the sources of stress have been identified, individuals can begin to incorporate a variety of stress-reduction techniques into their daily lives. These may include:

a. Relaxation practices: Mindfulness meditation, deep breathing exercises, yoga, or progressive muscle relaxation can help calm the mind and body.

b. Physical activity: Regular exercise, such as aerobic activities, strength training, or low-impact activities like walking, can help reduce stress and promote overall well-being.

c. Social engagement: Maintaining a strong social support network, whether through family, friends, or community groups, can provide a sense of connection and belonging that can buffer against the effects of stress.

d. Cognitive-behavioral strategies: Techniques like cognitive reframing, problem-solving, or journaling can help individuals develop a more balanced and resilient mindset in the face of stress.

e. Hobbies and leisure activities: Engaging in enjoyable hobbies, creative pursuits, or leisure activities can provide a much-needed respite from stress and contribute to a sense of fulfillment.

4. Seeking Professional Support

In some cases, individuals may benefit from seeking professional support to help manage chronic or debilitating stress. This may include:

a. Counseling or psychotherapy: Working with a mental health professional, such as a therapist or counselor, can provide valuable insights and strategies for coping with stress.

b. Stress management programs: Specialized programs or workshops focused on stress reduction and resilience-building can offer structured, evidence-based approaches to managing stress.

c. Integrative medicine approaches: Incorporating complementary therapies, such as acupuncture, massage, or biofeedback, can provide additional support for stress management.

Collaborating with healthcare providers can help ensure that individuals receive the appropriate level of support and guidance to effectively manage stress and its associated consequences.

Integrating Sleep and Stress Management into a Holistic Wellness Plan

Sleep and stress management are not isolated aspects of health; they are intricately connected and play a crucial role in an individual's overall well-being. By adopting a comprehensive, holistic approach to these interconnected domains, men over 50 can significantly improve their physical, mental, and emotional health.

1. Recognizing the Bidirectional Relationship

It's important to acknowledge the bidirectional relationship between sleep and stress. Poor sleep can contribute to increased stress levels, while chronic stress can also disrupt sleep patterns. Addressing these two elements in tandem is essential for achieving optimal outcomes.

2. Prioritizing a Balanced Lifestyle

Incorporating sleep and stress management strategies into a broader, balanced lifestyle plan can help men over 50 maintain a high quality of life and resilience in the face of the challenges that come with aging. This may include:

a. Maintaining a healthy, nutrient-dense diet
   b. Engaging in regular physical activity
   c. Cultivating meaningful social connections
   d. Pursuing intellectual stimulation and personal growth
   e. Practicing relaxation and mindfulness techniques

By addressing sleep, stress, and other key aspects of health in a comprehensive manner, individuals can create a solid foundation for overall well-being.

3. Collaborating with Healthcare Providers

Collaborating with healthcare professionals, such as primary care physicians, sleep specialists, mental health providers, or integrative medicine practitioners, is crucial for developing a personalized plan for optimizing sleep and managing stress. These experts can provide tailored guidance, recommend appropriate interventions, and monitor progress over time.

4. Embracing a Continuous Improvement Mindset

Improving sleep quality and effectively managing stress is an ongoing process, not a one-time event. Embracing a continuous improvement mindset, regularly monitoring progress, and being willing to adjust strategies as needed can help men over 50 navigate the dynamic nature of these health domains.

5. Fostering Resilience and Adaptability

Developing a resilient mindset and the ability to adapt to changing circumstances is crucial for effectively managing sleep and stress. By cultivating a positive outlook, practicing self-compassion, and embracing a problem-solving approach, individuals can better navigate the challenges that arise and maintain a high quality of life.

By integrating sleep and stress management into a comprehensive, holistic wellness plan, men over 50 can unlock a renewed sense of vitality, mental clarity, and emotional well-being, empowering them to thrive in the later stages of their lives.

Embracing the Journey of Sleep and Stress Mastery

Mastering sleep and stress management is not a simple task, but it is a critical investment in one's overall health and well-being. As men transition into their 50s, 60s, and beyond, prioritizing these two interconnected domains can have far-reaching benefits, from improving physical function and reducing the risk of chronic diseases to enhancing cognitive performance and emotional resilience.

Remember, the choices and strategies you implement today will lay the foundation for a more vibrant, resilient, and fulfilling future. Embrace the journey of sleep and stress mastery, collaborate with healthcare professionals, and trust that the steps you take will empower you to navigate the challenges of aging with confidence and grace.

By prioritizing sleep, managing stress, and incorporating these practices into a holistic wellness plan, men over 50 can unlock a renewed sense of purpose, vitality, and joy – the cornerstones of a truly meaningful and fulfilling life. Embrace this journey, and let it guide you towards a future filled with the energy, mental clarity, and emotional well-being that you deserve.

CHAPTER 8

P rioritizing Urological Health

As men transition into their later years, maintaining a healthy urological system becomes increasingly important. The aging process can bring about a variety of changes and challenges within the urinary tract and reproductive organs, requiring a proactive and comprehensive approach to address these often-overlooked aspects of men's health.

In this chapter, we will delve into the key urological concerns that men over 50 may face, from prostate health and urinary function to sexual well-being. We'll explore the underlying causes, the importance of early detection and management, and the strategies for preserving urological function and overall quality of life.

Understanding the Aging Urological System

The urological system, which includes the kidneys, ureters, bladder, and prostate gland, plays a crucial role in the body's waste elimination and reproductive functions. As men grow older, this complex system undergoes a series of physiological changes that can lead to a variety of health concerns.

1. Prostate Gland Changes
   One of the most prominent urological changes associated with aging is the gradual enlargement of the prostate gland, a condition known as benign

prostatic hyperplasia (BPH). The prostate, a walnut-sized gland located at the base of the bladder, plays a vital role in the male reproductive system, but its growth can lead to a variety of urinary symptoms as men age.

BPH can cause the prostate to compress the urethra, the tube that carries urine from the bladder out of the body, leading to difficulties with urination, such as a weak or interrupted stream, the need to urinate more frequently, and a feeling of incomplete bladder emptying.

2. Urinary Function Changes

In addition to prostate changes, the aging process can also affect the overall function of the urinary system. As men grow older, they may experience:

a. Decreased bladder capacity and control: The bladder can lose its ability to hold as much urine, leading to more frequent urination and potential incontinence.

b. Weakened bladder muscles: The muscles responsible for emptying the bladder may become weaker, making it more difficult to fully empty the bladder.

c. Increased risk of urinary tract infections: Older adults are more susceptible to developing urinary tract infections (UTIs) due to changes in the urinary tract and immune function.

3. Sexual Health Considerations

The urological system is closely linked to sexual function, and as men age, they may face a variety of challenges in this domain. These can include:

a. Erectile dysfunction: The gradual decline in testosterone production and other age-related changes can contribute to difficulties achieving and maintaining an erection.

b. Ejaculatory dysfunction: Older men may experience changes in the intensity or volume of ejaculation, as well as difficulties with ejaculatory control.

c. Fertility concerns: While fertility does not usually become a significant issue for older men, the gradual decline in sperm quality and quantity can make it more challenging to conceive children.

Understanding these age-related changes within the urological system is crucial for men over 50 to proactively address any emerging concerns and maintain optimal urological health.

Common Urological Conditions in Men After 50

As men navigate the later stages of life, they may face a variety of urological conditions that require attention and management. Recognizing the signs and symptoms of these common issues can help individuals seek timely medical care and implement appropriate interventions.

1. Benign Prostatic Hyperplasia (BPH)
   As mentioned earlier, BPH is one of the most prevalent urological conditions affecting men over 50. Symptoms of BPH may include:

- Difficulty starting or maintaining a steady stream of urine
    - Feeling of incomplete bladder emptying
    - Increased frequency and urgency of urination, particularly at night
    - Weak urine stream or intermittent flow
    - Straining or dribbling during urination

If left untreated, BPH can lead to more serious complications, such as kidney problems, urinary tract infections, or even bladder damage.

2. Prostate Cancer
   In addition to BPH, men over 50 also face an increased risk of developing prostate cancer, a condition characterized by the uncontrolled growth of cells within the prostate gland. Early-stage prostate cancer often does not produce any obvious symptoms, making regular screening and monitoring

essential for early detection and effective treatment.

Symptoms of more advanced prostate cancer may include:

- Difficulty starting or stopping the urine stream
    - Frequent or urgent need to urinate, especially at night
    - Blood in the urine or semen
    - Painful or difficult urination
    - Bone pain or discomfort

3. Erectile Dysfunction

Erectile dysfunction, the consistent inability to achieve or maintain an erection sufficient for satisfactory sexual activity, is a common concern for men as they age. Factors contributing to erectile dysfunction may include:

- Vascular health issues, such as atherosclerosis or high blood pressure
    - Hormonal imbalances, particularly a decline in testosterone
    - Neurological conditions, like Parkinson's disease or multiple sclerosis
    - Psychological factors, such as stress, anxiety, or depression

4. Urinary Incontinence

Urinary incontinence, the involuntary leakage of urine, can be a source of significant distress and impact an individual's quality of life. Common types of incontinence in older men include:

- Stress incontinence: Leakage of urine during physical activity, coughing, or sneezing
    - Urge incontinence: Sudden, uncontrollable urges to urinate
    - Mixed incontinence: A combination of stress and urge incontinence

Underlying causes of incontinence may include weakened pelvic floor muscles, prostate issues, neurological conditions, or certain medications.

5. Urinary Tract Infections (UTIs)

Older adults, including men over 50, are more susceptible to developing urinary tract infections, which can lead to symptoms such as:

- Frequent or urgent need to urinate
  - Burning or pain during urination
  - Blood in the urine
  - Lower abdominal discomfort or pain

Untreated UTIs can potentially spread to the kidneys and cause more serious health problems, emphasizing the importance of prompt diagnosis and appropriate treatment.

Recognizing these common urological conditions and seeking timely medical attention is crucial for men over 50 to maintain optimal urological health and prevent the development of more severe complications.

Proactive Strategies for Urological Health

Maintaining a proactive and comprehensive approach to urological health is essential for men over 50. By incorporating a range of strategies, individuals can effectively manage existing conditions, reduce the risk of developing new issues, and preserve their overall quality of life.

1. Regular Prostate Screenings

Regular prostate screenings, including digital rectal examinations and prostate-specific antigen (PSA) blood tests, are crucial for the early detection and management of prostate-related conditions, such as BPH and prostate cancer.

The American Urological Association recommends that men over 40 discuss the risks and benefits of prostate cancer screening with their healthcare providers and make an informed decision about the appropriate screening schedule based on their individual risk factors and preferences.

2. Maintaining Pelvic Floor Health

Strengthening the pelvic floor muscles, which support the bladder, urethra, and other urological structures, can help prevent or manage issues like urinary incontinence and erectile dysfunction.

Incorporating pelvic floor exercises, such as Kegel exercises, into a regular fitness routine can help improve urinary control and sexual function. Working with a pelvic floor physical therapist can also provide personalized guidance and support.

3. Lifestyle Modifications

Adopting certain lifestyle changes can have a positive impact on urological health. These may include:

a. Maintaining a healthy weight: Excess weight can contribute to the development of various urological conditions, including BPH and erectile dysfunction.

b. Quitting smoking: Smoking is a risk factor for several urological issues, including bladder cancer and erectile dysfunction.

c. Limiting alcohol consumption: Excessive alcohol intake can irritate the bladder and worsen urinary symptoms.

d. Staying hydrated: Drinking adequate amounts of water can help reduce the risk of urinary tract infections and support overall urinary tract function.

4. Medication Management

In some cases, healthcare providers may prescribe medications to help manage specific urological conditions, such as:

a. BPH: Medications like alpha-blockers or 5-alpha reductase inhibitors can help alleviate the symptoms of an enlarged prostate.

b. Erectile dysfunction: Oral medications, such as phosphodiesterase type

5 (PDE5) inhibitors, can improve erectile function.

   c. Overactive bladder: Anticholinergic or beta-3 agonist medications can help reduce the urge to urinate and improve bladder control.

It's essential to work closely with healthcare providers to ensure appropriate medication use and to monitor for any potential side effects.

5. Surgical Interventions

   In more severe or treatment-resistant cases, healthcare providers may recommend surgical interventions to address urological conditions. These may include:

a. Transurethral resection of the prostate (TURP): A minimally invasive procedure to remove excess prostate tissue and relieve BPH symptoms.

   b. Penile implants: For the treatment of severe or refractory erectile dysfunction, penile implants can restore sexual function.

   c. Incontinence surgery: Procedures like slings or artificial sphincters can help manage persistent urinary incontinence.

While surgery should be considered a last resort, it can be a highly effective option for managing certain urological conditions when conservative treatments have been exhausted.

Integrating Urological Health into a Comprehensive Wellness Plan

Prioritizing urological health is not just about addressing specific conditions; it is a critical component of an individual's overall well-being. By integrating urological health into a comprehensive wellness plan, men over 50 can ensure that this often-overlooked aspect of their health is adequately addressed and supported.

1. Collaboration with Healthcare Providers

   Establishing a strong partnership with healthcare providers, such as urologists, primary care physicians, and other specialists, is essential for developing and implementing an effective urological health plan. These professionals can provide personalized guidance, order necessary screenings and diagnostic tests, and collaborate on the most appropriate treatment strategies.

2. Regular Check-ups and Preventive Care

Consistent engagement in preventive care, including regular check-ups, prostate screenings, and routine monitoring of urological function, can help identify issues early and facilitate timely intervention. Men over 50 should work with their healthcare team to establish a personalized schedule for these screenings and assessments.

3. Holistic Approach to Sexual Health

Addressing urological concerns, such as erectile dysfunction or ejaculatory issues, should be part of a broader, holistic approach to sexual health. This may involve addressing underlying physical or psychological factors, as well as exploring strategies to maintain intimacy and a fulfilling sex life.

4. Integration with Other Health Domains

Urological health is closely connected to various other aspects of an individual's overall well-being, including cardiovascular health, hormonal balance, and mental/emotional wellness. Integrating urological care into a comprehensive health plan can help ensure that all these interconnected domains are adequately addressed and supported.

5. Empowerment Through Education and Self-Advocacy

Educating oneself about urological conditions, treatment options, and available resources is crucial for men over 50 to become active participants in their own healthcare. By empowering themselves through knowledge, individuals can make informed decisions, advocate for their needs, and play a more significant role in maintaining their urological health.

By embracing a holistic, proactive, and collaborative approach to urological health, men over 50 can safeguard this essential aspect of their well-being and enhance their overall quality of life.

Embracing the Journey of Urological Wellness

Maintaining a healthy urological system is a critical component of a man's overall health and well-being, particularly as he transitions into the later stages of life. By understanding the age-related changes within the urological system, addressing common conditions proactively, and integrating urological care into a comprehensive wellness plan, men over 50 can take control of this often-overlooked aspect of their health.

Remember, urological health is not just about managing specific conditions; it is about preserving your independence, maintaining your quality of life, and empowering yourself to live a fulfilling, vibrant existence. By prioritizing urological wellness, you can ensure that you have the physical and sexual function necessary to continue enjoying the activities, relationships, and experiences that bring you joy and purpose.

Embrace the journey of urological wellness, collaborate with your healthcare team, and trust that the steps you take today will pave the way for a future filled with confidence, comfort, and the ability to fully engage in life's most meaningful moments. Your urological health is a crucial investment in your overall well-being, and the dividends it can pay are invaluable.

CHAPTER 9

Navigating Sexual Health Challenges

As men transition into their later years, maintaining a healthy and fulfilling sex life can become a more complex and nuanced endeavor. The aging process can bring about various physiological, psychological, and relational changes that can impact sexual function, intimacy, and overall sexual well-being.

In this chapter, we will explore the unique sexual health considerations that men over 50 may face, delving into the underlying causes, the common challenges, and the strategies for addressing them effectively. By adopting a holistic and proactive approach to sexual health, individuals can preserve their intimate relationships, enhance their quality of life, and navigate the changes of aging with confidence and resilience.

Understanding the Aging Male Sexual System

The human sexual response is a complex, multifaceted process that involves a delicate interplay of physiological, psychological, and relational factors. As men grow older, these various components can undergo significant changes, which can impact their sexual function and overall sexual well-being.

1. Physiological Changes
    The aging process can bring about a variety of physiological changes that

can affect sexual function, including:

a. Hormonal shifts: The gradual decline in testosterone production, which begins around the age of 30, can lead to decreased libido, erectile dysfunction, and changes in sexual response.

b. Vascular health: Underlying cardiovascular conditions, such as atherosclerosis or hypertension, can impair blood flow to the penis, making it more difficult to achieve and maintain erections.

c. Neurological functioning: Certain neurological conditions, like Parkinson's disease or multiple sclerosis, can impact the neural pathways involved in sexual response and function.

d. Anatomical changes: The prostate gland may undergo enlargement (benign prostatic hyperplasia), potentially leading to urinary and sexual function issues.

2. Psychological and Relational Factors

In addition to the physiological changes, the aging process can also introduce psychological and relational factors that can impact sexual well-being, such as:

a. Body image and self-esteem: As men grow older, they may experience changes in their physical appearance and sexual performance, which can affect their self-confidence and body image.

b. Relationship dynamics: Shifts in long-term relationships, such as the loss of a partner or changes in intimacy, can significantly impact sexual function and satisfaction.

c. Mental health concerns: Conditions like depression, anxiety, or cognitive decline can interfere with desire, arousal, and overall sexual enjoyment.

d. Societal and cultural perceptions: Outdated societal attitudes and stigmas surrounding aging and sexuality can create additional barriers and challenges for men over 50.

Understanding the multifaceted nature of sexual health and the specific changes associated with aging is crucial for men to develop an effective strategy for maintaining a fulfilling and satisfying sex life.

Common Sexual Health Challenges in Men After 50

As men navigate the later stages of life, they may encounter a variety of sexual health challenges that can impact their intimate relationships and overall quality of life. Recognizing and addressing these issues proactively can help individuals preserve their sexual well-being and enhance their overall sense of fulfillment.

1. Erectile Dysfunction
   Erectile dysfunction, the persistent inability to achieve or maintain an erection sufficient for satisfactory sexual activity, is one of the most prevalent sexual health concerns for men over 50. This condition can have a variety of underlying causes, including:

- Vascular health issues, such as atherosclerosis or high blood pressure
    - Hormonal imbalances, particularly a decline in testosterone
    - Neurological conditions, like Parkinson's disease or multiple sclerosis
    - Psychological factors, such as stress, anxiety, or depression

Effectively managing erectile dysfunction often requires a multifaceted approach, involving lifestyle modifications, medication, and in some cases, medical interventions.

2. Decreased Libido
   As men age, they may experience a gradual decline in sexual desire or libido. This can be attributed to a combination of physiological, psychological, and relational factors, including:

- Hormonal changes, particularly the decrease in testosterone production
    - Underlying health conditions, such as cardiovascular disease or depres-

sion
- Relationship challenges or the loss of a partner
- Stress, fatigue, or changes in overall life priorities

Addressing decreased libido often involves a comprehensive approach that addresses the underlying causes and promotes overall sexual well-being.

3. Ejaculatory Dysfunction
Older men may also experience changes in their ejaculatory function, which can include:

- Delayed or diminished ejaculation
- Retrograde ejaculation (ejaculation into the bladder)
- Reduced ejaculatory volume or force

These issues can be influenced by a variety of factors, including prostate enlargement, nerve damage, or certain medications.

4. Prostate Health Concerns
As mentioned in the previous chapter, the aging process can lead to prostate gland enlargement (benign prostatic hyperplasia) or the development of prostate cancer, both of which can have a significant impact on sexual function. Symptoms may include pain, difficulty with urination, and changes in sexual performance.

5. Relationship and Intimacy Challenges
The aging process can also introduce complex relational and emotional challenges that can impact sexual well-being. These may include:

- Changing dynamics and intimacy within long-term relationships
- Grief and loss associated with the death of a partner
- Difficulty communicating about sexual needs and desires
- Societal stigmas and misconceptions surrounding aging and sexuality

Addressing these interpersonal and emotional factors is crucial for maintaining a fulfilling and satisfying sex life.

Recognizing these common sexual health challenges and seeking timely medical attention or professional support can help men over 50 take proactive steps to address and manage these issues effectively.

Strategies for Enhancing Sexual Well-Being

Maintaining a healthy and fulfilling sex life as men grow older requires a comprehensive, multifaceted approach that addresses the physical, psychological, and relational aspects of sexual well-being. By incorporating the following strategies, individuals can preserve their intimate relationships, enhance their quality of life, and navigate the changes of aging with confidence and resilience.

1. Addressing Underlying Health Conditions
Treating any underlying physical or medical conditions that may be contributing to sexual health challenges is a crucial first step. This may involve:

a. Managing cardiovascular health: Treating conditions like hypertension, high cholesterol, or atherosclerosis can help improve blood flow and sexual function.

b. Optimizing hormone levels: Addressing any imbalances in testosterone or other hormones through medication or lifestyle changes can positively impact sexual desire and function.

c. Managing neurological conditions: Addressing issues like Parkinson's disease or multiple sclerosis can help mitigate the impact on sexual response and function.

d. Addressing prostate health concerns: Effectively managing benign prostatic hyperplasia or prostate cancer can help preserve sexual and urinary function.

2. Incorporating Lifestyle Modifications

Adopting a healthy lifestyle can have a significant impact on sexual well-being. Strategies may include:

a. Maintaining a balanced diet: Consuming a nutrient-rich diet can support overall health and sexual function.

b. Engaging in regular exercise: Physical activity can improve cardiovascular health, boost mood, and enhance sexual performance.

c. Prioritizing stress management: Implementing stress-reduction techniques, such as meditation or relaxation practices, can help mitigate the negative effects of stress on sexual function.

d. Avoiding or limiting alcohol and tobacco use: Excessive consumption of these substances can impair sexual function and overall health.

3. Exploring Medications and Medical Interventions

In some cases, healthcare providers may recommend medications or medical interventions to address specific sexual health challenges, such as:

a. Oral medications for erectile dysfunction: Phosphodiesterase type 5 (PDE5) inhibitors, like sildenafil (Viagra) or tadalafil (Cialis), can help improve erectile function.

b. Hormone replacement therapy: Testosterone replacement therapy may be prescribed to address low libido or other sexual function issues related to hormonal changes.

c. Vacuum devices or penile implants: For more severe cases of erectile dysfunction, medical devices or surgical interventions may be considered.

It's important to work closely with healthcare providers to determine the most appropriate and effective treatment options.

4. Enhancing Intimacy and Communication

Addressing the psychological, emotional, and relational aspects of sexual well-being is equally important. Strategies may include:

a. Engaging in couples counseling or sex therapy: Working with a qualified therapist can help couples navigate changes in their intimate relationships and improve communication around sexual needs and desires.

b. Practicing mindfulness and body acceptance: Cultivating a positive self-image and being present during intimate moments can enhance sexual enjoyment and satisfaction.

c. Exploring new forms of intimacy: Adapting to changes in sexual function and finding alternative ways to express and experience intimacy can help maintain a fulfilling sex life.

d. Seeking support from peers or community resources: Connecting with support groups or educational resources can help men over 50 feel less isolated and more empowered in addressing sexual health challenges.

5. Embracing a Holistic Approach

Maintaining a holistic, comprehensive approach to sexual well-being is crucial for men over 50. This may involve:

a. Addressing interconnected health domains: Ensuring that other aspects of health, such as cardiovascular, hormonal, and mental health, are also optimized can have a positive impact on sexual function.

b. Collaborating with a multidisciplinary team: Working with healthcare providers from various disciplines, including primary care physicians, urologists, sex therapists, and mental health professionals, can provide a more comprehensive and personalized plan of care.

c. Prioritizing overall quality of life: Addressing sexual health challenges within the broader context of an individual's overall well-being, fulfillment, and life satisfaction can help ensure a more holistic and sustainable approach to sexual wellness.

By incorporating these strategies and embracing a holistic, proactive approach to sexual health, men over 50 can navigate the changes of aging with confidence, preserve their intimate relationships, and enhance their overall quality of life.

Addressing the Societal Stigma Around Aging and Sexuality

One of the significant barriers to maintaining a healthy and fulfilling sex life as men grow older is the pervasive societal stigma surrounding aging and sexuality. Outdated and often inaccurate beliefs and attitudes can create additional challenges for individuals seeking to address their sexual health concerns.

1. Confronting Misconceptions and Stereotypes

Many societal perceptions of aging and sexuality are rooted in misconceptions and outdated stereotypes, such as the idea that older adults are no longer interested in or capable of engaging in sexual activity. Challenging these beliefs and promoting a more inclusive, sex-positive narrative is crucial for empowering men over 50 to prioritize their sexual well-being.

2. Promoting Open Dialogue and Education

Fostering open and honest discussions about the realities of aging and sexuality can help destigmatize the topic and empower individuals to seek the support and resources they need. This may involve:

a. Encouraging healthcare providers to initiate conversations about sexual health with their older patients
b. Developing educational campaigns and resources that normalize the experience of aging and sexuality
c. Promoting peer-to-peer support and sharing of personal experiences to reduce feelings of isolation

3. Advocating for Age-Inclusive Representation

Ensuring that the media, marketing, and cultural narratives around sexuality and intimacy are inclusive of older adults can help challenge the prevailing societal biases. Increased representation of diverse, age-inclusive stories and images can help normalize and celebrate the sexual well-being of men over 50.

4. Empowering Individuals to Self-Advocate

Providing men over 50 with the tools and confidence to advocate for their sexual health needs can help them navigate the healthcare system, communicate with their partners, and address any societal stigmas they may encounter. This may involve:

a. Offering resources and guidance on how to discuss sexual health concerns with healthcare providers

b. Providing strategies for effective communication and negotiation within intimate relationships

c. Fostering a sense of empowerment and self-advocacy in the face of societal biases or unsupportive attitudes

By addressing the societal stigma surrounding aging and sexuality, we can create an environment that empowers men over 50 to prioritize their sexual well-being, seek the necessary support and resources, and maintain fulfilling intimate relationships throughout the later stages of life.

Embracing the Journey of Sexual Wellness

Maintaining a healthy and satisfying sex life is a vital component of overall well-being, and it is a journey that must be embraced with intention, resilience, and a commitment to self-care. As men navigate the changes and challenges associated with aging, it is crucial to adopt a proactive and holistic approach to sexual health, addressing the physical, psychological, and relational aspects that contribute to a fulfilling intimate life.

Remember, the sexual well-being of men over 50 is not just about physical function; it is about preserving the deep connections, emotional intimacy, and sense of fulfillment that are essential for a high quality of life. By addressing sexual health challenges head-on and incorporating strategies to enhance sexual wellness, individuals can continue to thrive in their intimate relationships, discover newfound avenues of pleasure and connection, and maintain a strong sense of self-worth and confidence.

Embrace the journey of sexual wellness, collaborate with healthcare providers and trusted partners, and trust that the steps you take today will pave the way for a future filled with intimacy, pleasure, and a profound sense of connection. Your sexual health is a vital investment in your overall well-being, and the rewards it can bring are immeasurable.

CHAPTER 10

F ostering Emotional Well-being

As men transition into their later years, maintaining emotional well-being becomes increasingly crucial for their overall health and quality of life. The aging process can bring about a unique set of challenges, from navigating life changes and adjusting to new roles to coping with the loss of loved ones and managing chronic health conditions. Ensuring that emotional and mental health needs are addressed can significantly impact an individual's ability to thrive and find fulfillment in the later stages of life.

In this chapter, we will explore the key aspects of emotional well-being for men over 50, including the common emotional challenges they may face, the importance of building a strong support network, and the strategies for cultivating resilience, balance, and a positive outlook. By adopting a proactive and comprehensive approach to emotional wellness, individuals can unlock a renewed sense of purpose, contentment, and the ability to navigate the complexities of aging with grace and resilience.

Understanding the Emotional Landscape of Aging

The emotional experiences of men over 50 can be multifaceted and dynamic, influenced by a variety of factors, both internal and external. Recognizing the common emotional challenges and their underlying causes is the first step in developing effective strategies for maintaining mental and emotional well-being.

1. Life Transitions and Adjustments

As men progress through the later stages of life, they may face significant life transitions and adjustments that can impact their emotional state. These may include:

a. Retirement and the loss of professional identity
   b. Caregiving responsibilities for aging parents or spouses
   c. The empty nest phase as children become independent
   d. Changing roles and responsibilities within the family and community

These transitions can bring about feelings of uncertainty, loss of purpose, and the need to redefine one's sense of identity and place in the world.

2. Grief and Loss

The aging process often coincides with the loss of loved ones, whether it's the death of a spouse, close friends, or family members. Navigating the grieving process and adjusting to the absence of these significant relationships can be emotionally challenging and can contribute to feelings of loneliness, depression, and anxiety.

3. Health Concerns and Chronic Conditions

The onset or progression of chronic health conditions, such as cardiovascular disease, cancer, or cognitive decline, can also have a significant impact on emotional well-being. Coping with the physical and practical implications of these health issues, as well as the psychological toll, can be a source of stress, anxiety, and even depression.

4. Societal Perceptions and Stigmas

Outdated societal perceptions and stigmas surrounding aging can also contribute to emotional challenges for men over 50. Feelings of marginalization, loss of social status, or a perceived lack of value can negatively impact self-esteem, self-worth, and overall emotional well-being.

5. Changing Relationships and Intimacy

As men navigate the later stages of life, their intimate relationships and social connections may also undergo significant changes. Adjusting to evolving family dynamics, the loss of a partner, or changes in sexual and intimacy patterns can be emotionally taxing and can lead to feelings of isolation and disconnection.

Understanding these common emotional challenges and their underlying causes is crucial for men over 50 to develop effective strategies for maintaining and enhancing their emotional well-being.

Cultivating a Strong Support Network

One of the most powerful tools for fostering emotional well-being in the later stages of life is the development and maintenance of a robust support network. By surrounding themselves with a diverse array of social connections and sources of emotional support, men can build a foundation for resilience, contentment, and a greater sense of purpose.

1. Nurturing Relationships with Family and Friends

Maintaining and strengthening relationships with family members, close friends, and other loved ones can provide a vital source of emotional support, companionship, and a sense of belonging. Regular communication, shared activities, and the opportunity to lean on one another during challenging times can help mitigate feelings of loneliness and isolation.

2. Engaging in Community Involvement

Participating in community-based organizations, clubs, or volunteer activities can help men over 50 expand their social circles, develop new connections, and feel a sense of purpose and fulfillment. These engagements can provide opportunities for social interaction, intellectual stimulation, and the cultivation of a support network beyond immediate family and friends.

3. Seeking Professional Support

In some cases, individuals may benefit from seeking professional support, such as that provided by mental health counselors, therapists, or support groups. These resources can offer specialized guidance, coping strategies, and a safe space to process emotions and work through personal challenges.

4. Leveraging Technology for Connectivity

In the modern digital age, technology can also play a role in helping men over 50 maintain and strengthen their support networks. Platforms for video calls, social media, and online communities can facilitate long-distance connections, provide access to virtual support groups, and help alleviate feelings of isolation.

5. Fostering Intergenerational Relationships

Cultivating meaningful connections with individuals of different age groups, such as younger family members or mentees, can provide a sense of purpose, wisdom-sharing, and the opportunity to contribute to the lives of others. These intergenerational relationships can help counter feelings of marginalization and promote a sense of value and belonging.

By intentionally building and nurturing a diverse support network, men over 50 can create a foundation for emotional well-being, resilience, and a greater sense of purpose throughout the later stages of life.

Developing Emotional Resilience and Coping Strategies

Alongside the development of a strong support network, fostering emotional resilience and implementing effective coping strategies are essential for maintaining mental and emotional well-being in the face of the challenges that often accompany aging.

1. Cultivating a Positive Mindset

Adopting a positive, optimistic outlook can play a crucial role in an individual's emotional well-being. This may involve:

a. Practicing gratitude and focusing on the positive aspects of one's life
b. Challenging negative thought patterns and reframing challenges as opportunities for growth
c. Embracing a growth mindset and a willingness to adapt to changes

By cultivating a positive mindset, men over 50 can better navigate the emotional ups and downs of the aging process and maintain a sense of resilience and purpose.

2. Engaging in Stress Management Techniques

Effective stress management is crucial for maintaining emotional balance and well-being. Incorporating a range of stress-reduction strategies, such as mindfulness practices, deep breathing exercises, or relaxation techniques, can help individuals better cope with the emotional demands of aging.

3. Prioritizing Self-Care and Work-Life Balance

Ensuring a healthy work-life balance and prioritizing self-care activities can help men over 50 maintain emotional well-being. This may include:

a. Engaging in regular physical activity, which can have positive effects on mood and stress levels
b. Pursuing hobbies, creative pursuits, or leisure activities that bring a sense of enjoyment and fulfillment
c. Maintaining a balanced, nutritious diet that supports overall physical and mental health

By taking an active role in their self-care, individuals can enhance their emotional resilience and overall quality of life.

4. Developing Coping Mechanisms for Grief and Loss

Navigating the grieving process associated with the loss of loved ones can be a significant emotional challenge. Developing healthy coping mechanisms, such as:

a. Engaging in rituals or ceremonies to honor the memory of the deceased

b. Seeking support from grief counselors, support groups, or bereavement services

c. Allowing oneself to fully experience and express emotions in a healthy manner

can help individuals work through the grieving process and find a sense of acceptance and healing.

5. Embracing Lifelong Learning and Personal Growth

Continuous learning and personal growth can provide a sense of purpose, intellectual stimulation, and a buffer against the potential emotional challenges of aging. Engaging in activities such as:

a. Acquiring new skills or hobbies

b. Exploring educational opportunities, such as taking classes or attending lectures

c. Volunteering or mentoring others to share one's knowledge and experience

can help foster a sense of accomplishment, belonging, and emotional fulfillment.

By incorporating these strategies for cultivating emotional resilience and coping mechanisms, men over 50 can build a strong foundation for maintaining mental and emotional well-being throughout the later stages of life.

Addressing Mental Health Concerns

While emotional well-being is a broader concept that encompasses an individual's overall mental, emotional, and psychological state, it is important to acknowledge and address any specific mental health concerns that may arise as men transition into their later years.

1. Recognizing and Managing Depression

Depression is a common mental health challenge faced by older adults, and it can have a significant impact on an individual's quality of life, relationships, and overall well-being. Symptoms of depression in men over 50 may include:

a. Persistent feelings of sadness, hopelessness, or emptiness
    b. Loss of interest in activities once enjoyed
    c. Changes in sleep patterns, appetite, or energy levels
    d. Difficulty concentrating or making decisions
    e. Thoughts of suicide or self-harm

Seeking professional help, such as from a mental health therapist or counselor, and exploring treatment options like therapy or medication can be crucial for effectively managing depression.

2. Addressing Anxiety and Worry

Anxiety and persistent worries can also be common emotional challenges for men over 50, particularly in the face of life changes, health concerns, or financial uncertainties. Symptoms of anxiety may include:

a. Excessive, uncontrollable worry or fear
    b. Physical symptoms like rapid heartbeat, shortness of breath, or muscle tension
    c. Difficulty sleeping or concentrating
    d. Avoidance of certain situations or activities

Incorporating stress-reduction techniques, cognitive-behavioral therapy, and, in some cases, medication can help individuals manage and overcome anxiety.

3. Managing Cognitive Decline and Dementia

As discussed in a previous chapter, age-related cognitive changes and the onset of conditions like Alzheimer's disease or other forms of dementia can have a significant emotional impact on individuals and their loved ones. Addressing these cognitive challenges proactively and seeking support can help mitigate the emotional toll and maintain a sense of dignity and independence.

4. Substance Abuse and Addiction

Substance abuse, including the misuse of alcohol or prescription medications, can also be a concern for men over 50 and can have a detrimental impact on emotional well-being. Seeking professional help and engaging in addiction treatment programs can be crucial for addressing these issues and supporting long-term recovery.

5. Suicidal Ideation and Self-Harm

In some cases, men over 50 may experience suicidal thoughts or engage in self-harm behaviors, which can be an indicator of significant emotional distress. It is essential to take any signs of suicidal ideation or self-harm seriously and seek immediate professional help, such as contacting a suicide prevention hotline or crisis support service.

By recognizing the potential mental health challenges that can arise and taking proactive steps to address them, men over 50 can maintain their emotional well-being, preserve their quality of life, and access the necessary support and resources to navigate the complexities of aging with resilience and purpose.

Integrating Emotional Well-Being into a Holistic Health Plan

Emotional well-being is not a standalone aspect of an individual's overall health; it is intricately connected to various other domains, including physical, cognitive, and social health. By adopting a comprehensive, holistic approach to emotional wellness, men over 50 can create a foundation for a fulfilling, resilient, and purposeful life in their later years.

1. Aligning Emotional Well-Being with Physical Health

Maintaining physical health and well-being can have a direct impact on emotional and mental health, and vice versa. Incorporating strategies that address both physical and emotional needs, such as regular exercise, a balanced diet, and effective stress management, can help create a synergistic approach to overall wellness.

2. Integrating Emotional Wellness into Cognitive Health

The preservation of cognitive function and the prevention or management of age-related cognitive decline are closely linked to emotional well-being. Strategies that support both cognitive and emotional health, such as engaging in mentally stimulating activities, practicing mindfulness, and building a strong social support network, can help individuals thrive in their later years.

3. Fostering Emotional Wellness in Interpersonal Relationships

Maintaining and nurturing healthy interpersonal relationships can be a crucial component of emotional well-being. Strategies that enhance communication, intimacy, and social connection can help men over 50 feel supported, valued, and engaged within their personal and community-based relationships.

4. Collaborating with Healthcare Providers

Collaborating with a diverse team of healthcare providers, including primary care physicians, mental health professionals, geriatric specialists, and therapists, can help ensure that all aspects of emotional well-being are addressed in a comprehensive and personalized manner.

5. Embracing a Continuous Improvement Mindset

Emotional well-being is not a static state; it is a dynamic and evolving process. Embracing a continuous improvement mindset, regularly monitoring progress, and being willing to adjust strategies as needed can help men over 50 navigate the ebb and flow of emotional challenges and maintain a high level of well-being throughout the later stages of life.

By integrating emotional well-being into a holistic health plan, men over 50 can create a foundation for a fulfilling, resilient, and purposeful life in their later years, empowering them to thrive in the face of the unique challenges and opportunities that come with aging.

Embracing the Journey of Emotional Wellness

Fostering emotional well-being is a vital component of a comprehensive health and wellness plan for men over 50. By understanding the common emotional challenges associated with aging, cultivating a strong support network, and developing strategies for cultivating resilience and coping with stress, individuals can enhance their overall quality of life and unlock a renewed sense of purpose, contentment, and the ability to navigate the complexities of later life with grace and resilience.

Remember, the emotional well-being of men over 50 is not just about managing mental health concerns; it is about creating a foundation for a fulfilling, meaningful, and emotionally balanced existence. By prioritizing emotional wellness and integrating it into a holistic health plan, individuals can unlock a deeper sense of self-awareness, emotional intelligence, and the ability to navigate the ever-evolving landscape of aging with confidence and resilience.

Embrace the journey of emotional wellness, collaborate with healthcare providers and trusted support systems, and trust that the steps you take today will pave the way for a future filled with emotional fulfillment, strong interpersonal connections, and a profound sense of purpose. Your emotional well-being is a vital investment in your overall health and the quality of your later years, and the rewards it can bring are truly invaluable.

CHAPTER 11

Embracing a Healthy Lifestyle

As men transition into their later years, embracing a healthy lifestyle becomes increasingly crucial for maintaining overall well-being, preventing the onset of chronic conditions, and ensuring a high quality of life. The aging process brings about a unique set of physiological, cognitive, and emotional changes that require a proactive and comprehensive approach to health and wellness.

In this chapter, we will explore the key elements of a healthy lifestyle for men over 50, focusing on the importance of a balanced diet, the role of regular physical activity, and the strategies for integrating these components into a sustainable, long-term plan. By adopting a holistic, evidence-based approach to their health, individuals can unlock a renewed sense of vitality, resilience, and the ability to thrive in the later stages of life.

The Foundations of a Balanced Diet

Proper nutrition is the cornerstone of a healthy lifestyle, and as men grow older, their dietary needs and considerations evolve to address the unique challenges of aging. By incorporating a nutrient-dense, well-balanced diet, individuals can support their physical, cognitive, and emotional well-being.

1. Macronutrient Balance

As men transition into their 50s and beyond, their macronutrient (protein, carbohydrates, and fat) requirements may shift to support overall health and body composition. Key considerations include:

a. Protein intake: Maintaining adequate protein intake, from sources like lean meats, poultry, fish, eggs, and plant-based options, is crucial for preserving muscle mass and supporting immune function.

b. Complex carbohydrates: Prioritizing complex, fiber-rich carbohydrates, such as whole grains, fruits, and vegetables, can help regulate blood sugar levels and support digestive health.

c. Healthy fats: Incorporating healthy fats, including those found in nuts, seeds, avocados, and fatty fish, can provide essential nutrients and support heart, brain, and hormone health.

2. Nutrient-Dense Foods

Focusing on the consumption of nutrient-dense foods is essential for men over 50 to ensure they are getting the necessary vitamins, minerals, and antioxidants to support their overall well-being. These may include:

a. Fruits and vegetables: A variety of colorful produce provides a wide range of phytonutrients, fiber, and anti-inflammatory compounds.

b. Whole grains: Oats, quinoa, brown rice, and other whole grain options offer complex carbohydrates, fiber, and essential B vitamins.

c. Lean proteins: Poultry, fish, eggs, and plant-based protein sources, such as legumes, provide high-quality protein and support muscle health.

d. Dairy or dairy alternatives: Dairy products or fortified plant-based alternatives can help meet calcium and vitamin D requirements.

e. Nuts and seeds: These nutrient-dense foods offer healthy fats, protein, fiber, and a variety of vitamins and minerals.

3. Hydration and Fluid Intake

Maintaining proper hydration is crucial for overall health, as dehydration can lead to a range of issues, including fatigue, cognitive impairment, and increased risk of urinary tract infections. Men over 50 should aim to consume an adequate amount of water and other hydrating fluids throughout the day.

4. Dietary Modifications for Specific Conditions

In some cases, men over 50 may need to make specific dietary modifications to address or manage certain health conditions, such as:

a. Heart health: Reducing sodium intake and incorporating heart-healthy fats can support cardiovascular function.

b. Diabetes management: Controlling carbohydrate intake and monitoring blood sugar levels can help manage type 2 diabetes.

c. Bone health: Increasing calcium and vitamin D intake can help maintain strong bones and prevent osteoporosis.

d. Prostate health: Incorporating foods that may support prostate function, such as tomatoes and cruciferous vegetables, can be beneficial.

By adopting a balanced, nutrient-dense dietary approach, men over 50 can support their physical, cognitive, and emotional well-being, laying the foundation for a healthier and more fulfilling later life.

Embracing Regular Physical Activity

Regular physical activity is a crucial component of a healthy lifestyle for men over 50. Engaging in a well-rounded exercise regimen can provide a multitude of benefits, from improving cardiovascular health and maintaining muscle strength to enhancing cognitive function and boosting overall mood and energy levels.

1. Cardiovascular Exercise

Incorporating regular cardiovascular exercise, such as brisk walking, swimming, cycling, or jogging, can help improve heart health, reduce the risk of chronic diseases, and maintain a healthy body weight. Aim for at least 150 minutes of moderate-intensity or 75 minutes of vigorous-intensity aerobic activity per week.

2. Strength Training

Resistance or strength training exercises, such as weightlifting, bodyweight exercises, or the use of resistance bands, are essential for preserving muscle mass, bone density, and overall physical function as men age. Aim to incorporate strength training activities at least two to three times per week.

3. Flexibility and Balance Training

Maintaining flexibility and balance is crucial for preventing falls, reducing the risk of injury, and supporting overall mobility. Incorporating stretching, yoga, or Tai Chi into your routine can help improve range of motion, stability, and coordination.

4. Personalized Approach to Exercise

When designing an exercise plan, it's important to take into account individual factors, such as current fitness level, any existing health conditions, and personal preferences. Consulting with a healthcare provider or a qualified exercise professional can help ensure that the program is tailored to meet your specific needs and goals.

5. Gradual Progression and Consistency

Adopting a gradual, progressive approach to physical activity and maintaining consistency are key to achieving long-term success. Start with manageable exercises and gradually increase the intensity, duration, and frequency over time to avoid injury and promote sustainable habit formation.

By embracing regular physical activity as a core component of a healthy lifestyle, men over 50 can reap a wide range of benefits, including:

- Improved cardiovascular health and reduced risk of chronic diseases
    - Increased muscle strength, bone density, and physical function
    - Enhanced cognitive function and mood

- Better sleep quality and stress management
- Increased energy, vitality, and overall quality of life

Integrating Physical Activity and Nutrition into a Lifestyle Plan

Adopting a healthy lifestyle is not just about implementing individual strategies; it's about creating a comprehensive, integrated plan that addresses multiple aspects of well-being. By combining a balanced, nutrient-dense diet with regular physical activity, men over 50 can unlock a synergistic approach to their health and wellness.

1. Aligning Dietary and Exercise Goals

When developing a healthy lifestyle plan, it's essential to align your dietary and exercise goals to ensure maximum effectiveness and sustainability. For example, if your primary goal is to maintain a healthy body weight, you would want to focus on a calorie-controlled, nutrient-dense diet combined with a well-rounded exercise routine that includes both cardiovascular and strength-training components.

2. Prioritizing Nutrient Timing and Recovery

Carefully timing your nutrient intake around your physical activity can help support muscle recovery, improve exercise performance, and enhance overall health. This may involve strategies like consuming protein-rich meals after strength training or ensuring adequate hydration and carbohydrate intake before and during endurance activities.

3. Addressing Specific Health Conditions

For men over 50 with pre-existing health conditions, such as cardiovascular disease, diabetes, or joint issues, it's crucial to work closely with healthcare providers to develop a tailored lifestyle plan that addresses their unique needs. This may involve specific dietary modifications, targeted exercise programs, and the implementation of other supportive therapies or interventions.

4. Fostering Sustainable Habits

Creating sustainable, long-term healthy habits is the key to success. This may involve strategies like meal planning, scheduling exercise routines, and finding ways to make physical activity and nutritious eating enjoyable and integrated into your daily life.

5. Embracing a Holistic Approach

Recognizing the interconnectedness of various aspects of health is essential for a truly effective healthy lifestyle plan. By integrating physical, mental, emotional, and social well-being into your overall approach, you can create a synergistic and comprehensive strategy for optimal health and fulfillment.

6. Continuous Monitoring and Adjustment

Regularly monitoring your progress, adjusting your plan as needed, and being willing to adapt to changing circumstances are crucial for maintaining a healthy lifestyle in the long run. This may involve periodic check-ups with healthcare providers, tracking your biometrics, and being open to trying new approaches that better suit your evolving needs and preferences.

By adopting a comprehensive, integrated approach to a healthy lifestyle, men over 50 can unlock a renewed sense of vitality, resilience, and the ability to thrive in the later stages of life.

Overcoming Barriers and Challenges

Embracing a healthy lifestyle can be a rewarding and empowering journey, but it's not without its challenges. Men over 50 may face various barriers and obstacles that can hinder their efforts to adopt and maintain healthy habits. Understanding and addressing these challenges can help individuals overcome them and stay on track with their wellness goals.

1. Physical Limitations and Chronic Conditions

As men age, they may face physical limitations or the onset of chronic health conditions that can make adopting and maintaining a healthy lifestyle more difficult. Strategies to overcome these challenges may include:

- Working closely with healthcare providers to manage underlying conditions
    - Modifying exercise routines to accommodate physical limitations
    - Seeking guidance from exercise specialists or physical therapists
    - Gradually building up strength, flexibility, and endurance over time

2. Time Constraints and Competing Priorities
    The demands of work, family responsibilities, and other commitments can make it challenging for men over 50 to prioritize their health and wellness. Overcoming this barrier may involve:

- Scheduling and planning healthy activities and meals in advance
    - Seeking support from family members or caregivers
    - Identifying opportunities to integrate physical activity and healthy eating into daily routines
    - Learning to manage time effectively and set boundaries when necessary

3. Lack of Motivation and Habit Formation
    Maintaining the motivation and discipline to sustain healthy habits can be an ongoing challenge. Strategies to address this may include:

- Finding enjoyable, intrinsically motivated activities and pursuits
    - Enlisting the support of friends, family, or a accountability partner
    - Celebrating small wins and milestones along the way
    - Reframing setbacks as opportunities for growth and learning

4. Financial Considerations
    The costs associated with a healthy lifestyle, such as nutritious foods, gym memberships, or specialized healthcare, can be a barrier for some individuals. Addressing this challenge may involve:

- Exploring cost-effective options, such as community resources or online fitness programs
    - Prioritizing essential health investments and finding creative ways to save on other expenses
    - Seeking guidance from healthcare providers or financial advisors to manage health-related costs

5. Societal Perceptions and Stigmas

Outdated societal perceptions and stigmas surrounding aging can also present challenges for men over 50 who are attempting to adopt a healthy lifestyle. Addressing this may involve:

- Challenging negative stereotypes and promoting positive, age-inclusive narratives
    - Surrounding oneself with a supportive community that values health and wellness
    - Advocating for age-inclusive representation and resources in the health-care and fitness industries

By acknowledging and addressing these common barriers and challenges, men over 50 can develop strategies to overcome them and maintain a healthy lifestyle that supports their overall well-being and quality of life.

Embracing the Journey of Healthy Living

Embracing a healthy lifestyle is not a one-time event; it is a lifelong journey that requires dedication, flexibility, and a commitment to continuous improvement. As men transition into their later years, adopting a comprehensive, holistic approach to health and wellness can provide a solid foundation for a fulfilling, resilient, and empowered later life.

Remember, the choices you make today regarding your diet, physical activity, and overall wellness have a profound impact on your future. By prioritizing a healthy lifestyle, you are not only investing in your physical health but also supporting your cognitive, emotional, and social well-being – the key pillars of a truly rewarding and purposeful existence.

Embrace the journey of healthy living, collaborate with healthcare providers and trusted support systems, and trust that the steps you take today will pave the way for a future filled with vitality, resilience, and the ability to fully engage in the activities, relationships, and experiences that bring you joy and fulfillment. Your healthy lifestyle is a precious gift that you can cultivate and nurture, unlocking a world of possibilities in your later years.

CHAPTER 12

Staying Active and Independent

As men transition into their later years, maintaining physical function, mobility, and independence becomes an increasingly important aspect of overall health and well-being. The aging process can bring about a gradual decline in strength, flexibility, and balance, which can significantly impact an individual's ability to perform everyday tasks, engage in physical activities, and live autonomously.

In this chapter, we will explore the strategies and interventions that men over 50 can implement to preserve their physical capabilities, prevent falls and injuries, and adapt to the changes that come with aging. By adopting a proactive, comprehensive approach to maintaining an active and independent lifestyle, individuals can enhance their quality of life, reduce the risk of chronic health conditions, and continue to thrive in their later years.

Understanding the Physiological Changes of Aging

As men grow older, their bodies undergo a series of physiological changes that can impact their physical function and mobility. Recognizing these age-related alterations is the first step in developing an effective plan for preserving physical independence and active living.

1. Musculoskeletal Changes

One of the primary areas affected by the aging process is the musculoskeletal system. Men over 50 may experience:

a. Gradual loss of muscle mass and strength (sarcopenia)
  b. Decreased bone density and increased risk of osteoporosis
  c. Reduced flexibility and range of motion in joints
  d. Decreased balance and proprioception (awareness of body position)

These changes can contribute to a higher risk of falls, injuries, and a general decline in physical function and mobility.

2. Cardiovascular and Respiratory Changes

The cardiovascular and respiratory systems also undergo age-related changes that can impact physical performance and endurance. These may include:

a. Stiffening of blood vessels and reduced cardiovascular efficiency
  b. Decreased lung capacity and respiratory muscle strength
  c. Reduced exercise tolerance and increased fatigue during physical activity

These physiological alterations can make it more challenging for older adults to engage in physically demanding activities and maintain an active lifestyle.

3. Neurological Alterations

The aging process can also bring about changes within the nervous system, which can affect balance, coordination, and overall physical function. Examples include:

a. Reduced nerve conduction speed and sensory perception
  b. Slower reaction times and decreased responsiveness
  c. Potential development of neurological conditions, such as Parkinson's disease or peripheral neuropathy

These neurological changes can contribute to an increased risk of falls and difficulties with physical mobility and independence.

Understanding these physiological changes associated with aging is crucial for men over 50 to develop targeted strategies for maintaining physical function, preventing injuries, and adapting to the evolving needs of their bodies.

Maintaining Mobility and Preventing Falls

One of the primary goals for men over 50 is to maintain mobility, independence, and the ability to perform everyday tasks without assistance. Preventing falls and related injuries is a crucial aspect of this endeavor, as falls can have serious consequences and significantly impact an individual's quality of life.

1. Improving Strength and Balance
   Incorporating a well-rounded exercise routine that focuses on improving strength, balance, and coordination can be highly effective in maintaining physical function and reducing the risk of falls. This may include:

a. Resistance training to build and maintain muscle mass
   b. Balance exercises, such as standing on one leg or using a balance board
   c. Flexibility and stretching activities to improve range of motion
   d. Tai Chi or other mind-body exercises that challenge both physical and mental aspects of balance

Working with a qualified exercise professional, such as a physical therapist or personal trainer, can help men over 50 develop a personalized program that addresses their specific needs and abilities.

2. Optimizing Gait and Mobility
   Ensuring proper gait and mobility patterns can also play a significant role in fall prevention. Strategies may include:

a. Evaluating and addressing any underlying issues, such as joint pain or muscle imbalances, that may be affecting gait and mobility

b. Incorporating exercises and techniques to improve walking efficiency, stride length, and foot placement

c. Considering the use of assistive devices, such as canes or walkers, if needed to enhance stability and confidence during ambulation

3. Home Safety and Environmental Modifications

Assessing and addressing potential hazards within the home environment can help reduce the risk of falls. This may involve:

a. Removing tripping hazards, such as loose rugs or clutter

b. Ensuring adequate lighting, especially in high-traffic areas

c. Installing grab bars, railings, or non-slip surfaces in the bathroom

d. Considering the use of smart home technologies or mobility aids, like stair lifts or wheelchair ramps, if needed

4. Regular Physical Assessments and Intervention

Regularly evaluating physical function, balance, and fall risk through screenings and assessments can help identify any areas of concern and guide the development of targeted interventions. This may include:

a. Coordination with healthcare providers, such as physical therapists or occupational therapists, to conduct comprehensive assessments

b. Participation in structured fall prevention programs or balance training classes

c. Ongoing monitoring and adjustments to the individual's exercise routine or home environment modifications

By prioritizing the maintenance of strength, balance, and mobility, and taking proactive steps to address potential fall hazards, men over 50 can preserve their independence, reduce the risk of injuries, and continue to engage in the activities and pursuits they enjoy.

Adapting to Age-Related Physical Changes

While the aging process can bring about a gradual decline in physical function, men over 50 can adopt a range of strategies to adapt to these changes and maintain an active, independent lifestyle. By embracing a mindset of resilience and flexibility, individuals can overcome the challenges posed by age-related physical alterations.

1. Modifying Physical Activities

As men grow older, they may need to adapt or modify their physical activities to accommodate changes in strength, flexibility, and endurance. This may involve:

a. Transitioning from high-impact to low-impact exercises, such as swimming, cycling, or elliptical training

b. Incorporating more gentle, restorative exercises like yoga, Pilates, or tai chi

c. Adjusting the duration, intensity, and frequency of physical activities to match their current capabilities

By being open to trying new activities and finding ways to adapt existing pursuits, individuals can continue to enjoy an active lifestyle while managing the effects of aging.

2. Utilizing Assistive Devices and Technology

Incorporating assistive devices or leveraging technology can help men over 50 maintain their independence and continue engaging in physical activities and everyday tasks. Examples may include:

a. Mobility aids like canes, walkers, or wheelchairs to enhance stability and safety during ambulation

b. Ergonomic tools or adaptive equipment to make everyday tasks easier, such as reachers or grab bars

c. Smart home technologies that can monitor activity, detect falls, or provide remote assistance

By embracing these supportive tools, individuals can overcome physical limitations and preserve their autonomy.

3. Adapting Living Spaces and Environments

Modifying the home environment and other living spaces can also help men over 50 navigate the physical changes associated with aging. This may involve:

a. Implementing home renovations or accessibility upgrades, such as installing ramps, widening doorways, or lowering countertops

b. Reorganizing the home to prioritize accessibility and minimize the risk of falls or injuries

c. Exploring community resources or retirement living options that provide supportive, age-friendly environments

By creating a space that is tailored to their evolving needs, individuals can maintain a sense of independence and safety within their own homes.

4. Seeking Professional Support and Rehabilitation

In some cases, men over 50 may require specialized support or rehabilitation services to help them adapt to age-related physical changes. This may include:

a. Working with physical therapists or occupational therapists to develop personalized exercise programs and adaptive strategies

b. Participating in structured rehabilitation programs, such as those focused on fall prevention or functional mobility

c. Collaborating with healthcare providers to manage underlying health conditions that may be contributing to physical limitations

By proactively seeking professional guidance and support, individuals can develop effective strategies for maintaining their physical capabilities and independence.

5. Cultivating a Flexible, Resilient Mindset

Embracing a flexible, resilient mindset is crucial for successfully adapting to the physical changes associated with aging. This may involve:

a. Practicing self-compassion and avoiding self-criticism when faced with physical limitations

b. Maintaining a willingness to try new activities, adapt existing routines, and explore alternative solutions

c. Focusing on what one can still do, rather than lamenting over lost abilities

d. Seeking social support and engaging in activities that foster a sense of purpose and fulfillment

By adopting a flexible, adaptable approach, men over 50 can navigate the physical challenges of aging with greater resilience and a renewed sense of empowerment.

Integrating Physical Function and Independence into a Holistic Wellness Plan

Maintaining physical function and independence is not a standalone objective; it is an integral component of a comprehensive, holistic approach to health and well-being. By integrating these elements into a broader wellness plan, men over 50 can unlock a synergistic approach to their physical, mental, emotional, and social needs.

1. Aligning Physical Function with Other Health Domains

Preserving physical function and independence has implications for various other aspects of health, including:

a. Cognitive health: Maintaining physical activity and mobility can help support brain function and prevent cognitive decline.

b. Emotional well-being: The ability to remain physically active and independent can contribute to a greater sense of purpose, self-worth, and overall life satisfaction.

c. Social engagement: Maintaining physical function allows for continued participation in social activities and community involvement.

By recognizing these interconnections, individuals can develop a more comprehensive plan that addresses their holistic health needs.

2. Collaborating with Healthcare Providers

Collaborating with a team of healthcare providers, including primary care physicians, physical therapists, occupational therapists, and other specialists, is crucial for developing and implementing a personalized plan for maintaining physical function and independence. These professionals can provide tailored assessments, recommendations, and ongoing support.

3. Embracing a Proactive, Preventive Approach

Taking a proactive, preventive approach to physical function and independence is essential for men over 50. This may involve regular assessments, early intervention for any emerging issues, and the implementation of strategies to mitigate the risk of future decline.

4. Fostering Social Connections and Support Networks

Maintaining a strong social support network can play a vital role in preserving physical function and independence. Engaging in social activities, participating in community programs, and seeking the assistance of family and friends can enhance motivation, provide practical support, and foster a sense of purpose and belonging.

5. Continuous Monitoring and Adaptation

Regularly monitoring progress, identifying any changes or challenges, and being willing to adapt strategies as needed are crucial for maintaining physical function and independence over time. This flexibility and responsiveness to evolving needs can help ensure the long-term success of the wellness plan.

By integrating physical function and independence into a comprehensive, holistic approach to health and well-being, men over 50 can create a solid foundation for a fulfilling, autonomous, and resilient later life.

Embracing the Journey of Active, Independent Living

Maintaining physical function and independence is a vital component of a healthy, meaningful, and empowered later life. As men transition into their 50s, 60s, and beyond, embracing a proactive, adaptable, and comprehensive approach to preserving their physical capabilities can unlock a renewed sense of vitality, confidence, and the ability to continue engaging in the activities and pursuits that bring them joy and fulfillment.

Remember, the choices and strategies you implement today can have a profound impact on your future. By prioritizing the maintenance of strength, balance, and mobility, and adapting to the evolving needs of your body, you can ensure that you remain physically capable, independent, and empowered to navigate the challenges of aging with resilience and grace.

Embrace the journey of active, independent living, collaborate with health-care providers and supportive communities, and trust that the steps you take will pave the way for a future filled with autonomy, physical function, and the freedom to fully engage in the experiences that matter most to you. Your physical well-being is a precious gift that you can cultivate and nurture, unlocking a world of possibilities in your later years.

CHAPTER 13

Accessing Healthcare and Resources

As men navigate the later stages of life, navigating the complex healthcare system and accessing the necessary resources can become increasingly challenging. With a myriad of options, services, and support networks available, it is essential for individuals over 50 to develop a proactive and strategic approach to their healthcare needs.

In this chapter, we will explore the key elements of effectively accessing and utilizing the healthcare system, identifying and leveraging supportive community resources, and empowering men to take an active role in managing their well-being. By adopting a comprehensive and collaborative approach, individuals can ensure that they receive the appropriate care, support, and resources to thrive in their later years.

Navigating the Healthcare System Effectively

The healthcare system can be a daunting and fragmented landscape, particularly for older adults who may be dealing with multiple medical conditions or complex care needs. Understanding how to navigate this system and advocate for one's own healthcare interests is crucial for men over 50.

1. Establishing a Primary Care Relationship
   A primary care provider, such as a family medicine physician or an internist,

serves as the foundation of an individual's healthcare journey. Establishing a long-term relationship with a primary care provider can offer numerous benefits, including:

a. Coordinating comprehensive care and managing chronic conditions
b. Providing preventive screenings and health maintenance services
c. Serving as a trusted advisor and advocate within the healthcare system
d. Facilitating seamless transitions of care and referrals to specialists when needed

When selecting a primary care provider, men over 50 should consider factors such as the provider's experience, communication style, and commitment to patient-centered care.

2. Navigating the Specialist Network
As individuals age, they may require the expertise of various medical specialists, such as cardiologists, urologists, or geriatric specialists. Effectively navigating this network of specialists involves:

a. Obtaining referrals from the primary care provider to ensure appropriate and coordinated care
b. Researching and selecting specialists with experience in treating older adults and the specific conditions of concern
c. Maintaining open communication between the primary care provider and specialists to ensure a cohesive treatment approach
d. Advocating for the coordination of care among multiple providers to avoid fragmentation and duplication of services

3. Understanding Insurance Coverage and Costs
Navigating the complexities of health insurance can be a significant challenge for men over 50. Key considerations include:

a. Thoroughly understanding the coverage provided by Medicare, supplemental plans, or private insurance

b. Identifying any gaps or limitations in coverage and exploring options to fill those gaps

c. Researching and comparing the costs associated with different healthcare services, medications, and treatments

d. Seeking guidance from healthcare financial counselors or insurance specialists to optimize coverage and manage out-of-pocket expenses

4. Participating in Healthcare Decisions

Taking an active role in healthcare decision-making is crucial for men over 50 to ensure that their needs and preferences are met. This may involve:

a. Asking questions, voicing concerns, and collaborating with healthcare providers to develop personalized treatment plans

b. Advocating for second opinions or alternative treatment options when appropriate

c. Maintaining open and transparent communication with the healthcare team to promote shared decision-making

d. Utilizing patient portals, telehealth services, or other technologies to stay informed and engaged in their care

By developing a comprehensive understanding of the healthcare system and learning to navigate it effectively, men over 50 can take a more proactive and empowered approach to their well-being.

Identifying and Accessing Community Resources

In addition to navigating the healthcare system, men over 50 can benefit from identifying and utilizing a wide range of community-based resources and support services. These resources can complement and enhance the care received through the formal healthcare system, providing a holistic approach to meeting their needs.

1. Local and Regional Support Services

Exploring local and regional support services can offer a wealth of resources for men over 50. These may include:

a. Senior centers or community centers that provide social activities, educational programs, and wellness classes

b. Meal delivery or transportation services to help maintain independence and access essential resources

c. Support groups or counseling services for addressing mental health, grief, or caregiver-related challenges

d. Home modification or assistive technology programs to enhance safety and accessibility within the home

2. National and Online Resources

In addition to local resources, there are a variety of national and online resources that can benefit men over 50, such as:

a. Government-sponsored programs like Medicare, Medicaid, or the Department of Veterans Affairs

b. Non-profit organizations focused on specific health conditions or aging-related issues

c. Online communities, discussion forums, and educational platforms that provide information and peer support

d. Telehealth services or mobile applications that offer remote access to healthcare providers and wellness resources

3. Financial and Legal Assistance

Navigating the financial and legal aspects of aging can be complex, and accessing the appropriate resources and guidance is crucial. Examples include:

a. Financial planning services, such as retirement advisors or elder law attorneys

b. Tax preparation assistance, including programs that offer free or low-cost tax filing services for older adults

c. Benefit eligibility and enrollment support, including help with navigating Medicare, Medicaid, or other government-sponsored programs

d. Estate planning services, such as creating wills, powers of attorney, or advanced directives

4. Caregiver Support and Respite Services

For men over 50 who are caring for aging spouses, parents, or other loved ones, accessing caregiver support and respite services can be invaluable. These resources may include:

a. Respite care services, such as in-home care or adult day programs, to provide temporary relief for caregivers

b. Support groups, counseling, or educational programs specifically designed for family caregivers

c. Referrals to home healthcare agencies, assisted living facilities, or long-term care options when needed

d. Guidance on navigating the complex caregiving landscape and accessing relevant community resources

By identifying and leveraging the diverse array of community resources available, men over 50 can supplement the care they receive from the healthcare system, address their holistic needs, and maintain a high quality of life as they age.

Empowering Individuals to Take an Active Role

Ultimately, the most effective approach to accessing healthcare and community resources involves empowering men over 50 to take an active and engaged role in managing their well-being. By fostering self-advocacy, health literacy, and a collaborative mindset, individuals can optimize their healthcare experiences and ensure that their needs are met.

1. Promoting Health Literacy

Improving health literacy, or the ability to understand and make informed decisions about one's health, is a critical component of empowerment. Strategies to enhance health literacy may include:

a. Encouraging individuals to ask questions, voice concerns, and actively participate in their care

b. Providing educational resources and materials that help men over 50 understand their health conditions, treatment options, and available resources

c. Collaborating with healthcare providers to ensure clear communication and the use of easy-to-understand language

d. Fostering the development of personal health management skills, such as medication adherence, symptom monitoring, and self-care techniques

2. Cultivating Self-Advocacy Skills

Developing self-advocacy skills enables men over 50 to effectively navigate the healthcare system and advocate for their own needs. This may involve:

a. Encouraging individuals to be proactive in seeking out information, expressing preferences, and making informed decisions

b. Providing guidance on how to effectively communicate with healthcare providers, request second opinions, or challenge treatment recommendations when necessary

c. Empowering individuals to assert their rights, such as the right to access their medical records or the right to receive clear explanations of their care plan

d. Fostering the confidence and resilience to persist in the face of challenges or barriers within the healthcare system

3. Facilitating Collaborative Partnerships

Promoting a collaborative partnership between individuals and their healthcare providers is essential for ensuring that the unique needs and preferences of men over 50 are met. Strategies to foster this collaboration may include:

a. Encouraging open and transparent communication between individuals and their healthcare team

b. Facilitating the development of shared decision-making processes, where providers and patients work together to determine the most appropriate course of action

c. Promoting the use of patient-reported outcome measures to capture the individual's perspective on their health and well-being

d. Connecting individuals with resources and support services that can help them become active participants in their care

4. Leveraging Technology and Digital Tools

Incorporating technology and digital tools can empower men over 50 to take a more active role in managing their healthcare. Examples may include:

a. Utilization of patient portals or mobile applications to access medical records, communicate with providers, and schedule appointments

b. Engagement in telehealth services, which can improve access to healthcare and facilitate remote monitoring of health conditions

c. Adoption of wearable devices or home-based monitoring systems to track vital signs, physical activity, and other health metrics

d. Participation in online communities or educational platforms that provide information, support, and resources

By empowering men over 50 to take an active and engaged role in their healthcare, we can help ensure that they receive the appropriate care, support, and resources to thrive in their later years.

Integrating Healthcare and Community Resources into a Holistic Wellness Plan

Navigating the healthcare system and accessing community resources are not isolated endeavors; they are integral components of a comprehensive, holistic approach to well-being. By integrating these elements into a broader wellness plan, men over 50 can create a cohesive and synergistic strategy for maintaining their health, independence, and quality of life.

1. Aligning Healthcare Needs with Overall Wellness Goals

When developing a holistic wellness plan, it is essential to ensure that the healthcare and community resources being accessed are aligned with the individual's overall health and wellness goals. This may involve:

a. Identifying the specific health conditions, preventive care needs, and functional capabilities that must be addressed

b. Determining how community-based resources can complement and enhance the care received through the healthcare system

c. Integrating the various healthcare providers, specialists, and community support services into a coordinated plan of action

2. Fostering Collaborative Relationships with Healthcare Providers

Building strong, collaborative relationships with healthcare providers is crucial for the successful integration of healthcare and community resources. This may include:

a. Encouraging open communication and shared decision-making between individuals and their healthcare team

b. Facilitating the coordination of care among multiple providers to ensure a cohesive and comprehensive approach

c. Empowering individuals to advocate for their needs and preferences within the healthcare system

3. Leveraging Community Resources to Support Holistic Wellness

Community-based resources can play a vital role in supporting the various aspects of an individual's holistic wellness plan. This may involve:

a. Utilizing social and recreational programs to enhance emotional well-being and social engagement

b. Accessing financial planning or legal services to ensure the long-term security and stability of the individual's overall well-being

c. Engaging with caregiver support services or respite care options to maintain the individual's independence and quality of life

4. Continuous Monitoring and Adaptation

Regularly reviewing and adapting the holistic wellness plan is essential to ensure that it remains relevant and effective over time. This may include:

a. Monitoring the individual's progress, identifying any changes in needs or preferences, and making adjustments accordingly

b. Staying up-to-date with the evolving landscape of healthcare and community resources, and incorporating new options as they become available

c. Fostering a collaborative partnership with healthcare providers and community organizations to ensure a coordinated and responsive approach to the individual's well-being

By integrating healthcare and community resources into a comprehensive, holistic wellness plan, men over 50 can create a robust and adaptable framework for maintaining their health, independence, and quality of life throughout the later stages of their lives.

Embracing the Journey of Empowered Healthcare Navigation

Navigating the healthcare system and accessing the necessary resources can be a complex and daunting task, but it is a crucial component of a fulfilling and empowered later life. By developing a proactive, strategic, and collaborative approach to their healthcare and community-based support, men over 50 can ensure that their unique needs and preferences are met, and that they can continue to thrive and enjoy a high quality of life.

Remember, your healthcare journey is not something you must navigate alone. By embracing a mindset of self-advocacy, health literacy, and collaborative partnership with your healthcare providers and community resources, you can take an active and empowered role in managing your well-being. The choices you make today can have a profound impact on your future, so it is essential to prioritize your healthcare needs and access the support and resources that will enable you to live your best life.

Embrace the journey of empowered healthcare navigation, collaborate with your healthcare team and community partners, and trust that the steps you take will pave the way for a future filled with optimal health, independence, and the ability to fully engage in the experiences and relationships that bring you joy and fulfillment. Your healthcare is a precious investment in your overall well-being, and the dividends it can pay are truly invaluable.

CHAPTER 14

Inspiring a Fulfilling Retirement

As men transition into the later stages of life, the retirement years can present a unique set of opportunities and challenges. No longer bound by the demands of full-time employment, individuals have the chance to redefine their priorities, explore new hobbies and interests, and embark on the next chapter of their lives with a renewed sense of purpose and fulfillment.

In this chapter, we will explore the strategies and considerations for navigating the retirement journey, from the practical aspects of financial planning and healthcare management to the emotional and psychological factors that can contribute to a rewarding and meaningful retirement. By adopting a proactive and comprehensive approach, men over 50 can unlock a future filled with personal growth, adventure, and a deep sense of well-being.

Transitioning to Retirement with Purpose

The transition to retirement can be both an exciting and daunting prospect, as individuals grapple with the shift in their daily routines, social connections, and sense of identity. Approaching this transition with intentionality and a clear vision for the future can help men over 50 navigate this pivotal life stage with confidence and purpose.

1. Redefining Your Sense of Purpose

One of the primary challenges that can arise during retirement is the loss of a clear sense of purpose and direction. After years of being defined by their careers, many men struggle to find new avenues for personal fulfillment and meaningful contribution. Strategies for redefining purpose in retirement may include:

a. Exploring new hobbies, interests, or volunteer work that align with your values and passions

b. Engaging in lifelong learning opportunities, such as taking classes or pursuing new skills

c. Mentoring or sharing your expertise with younger generations

d. Prioritizing relationships and deepening connections with family, friends, and community

By proactively cultivating a sense of purpose, individuals can unlock a renewed zest for life and a greater sense of personal satisfaction in their retirement years.

2. Managing the Psychological Transition

The psychological and emotional aspects of transitioning to retirement can be just as significant as the practical considerations. Men over 50 may experience a range of emotions, including:

a. Feelings of loss or uncertainty about their new identity and role

b. Challenges in adjusting to a more unstructured daily routine

c. Concerns about maintaining social connections and avoiding isolation

d. Anxiety or apprehension about financial security and healthcare management

Addressing these psychological factors through strategies like counseling, support groups, or mindfulness practices can help facilitate a smoother and more fulfilling transition to retirement.

3. Developing a Retirement Roadmap

Creating a comprehensive retirement roadmap can provide a sense of structure, clarity, and direction during this significant life change. This may involve:

a. Outlining your short-term and long-term goals, interests, and lifestyle preferences

b. Mapping out a plan for managing your finances, healthcare, and daily activities

c. Identifying resources and support systems that can help you navigate the retirement journey

d. Regularly reviewing and adjusting your roadmap to accommodate evolving needs and preferences

By proactively planning for retirement, individuals can feel empowered and better equipped to embrace the opportunities and overcome the challenges that may arise.

Embracing New Hobbies and Opportunities

One of the most exciting aspects of retirement is the opportunity to explore new hobbies, interests, and activities that may have been put on the back burner during the demands of full-time work. Embracing these new experiences can provide a sense of fulfillment, personal growth, and enhanced well-being.

1. Discovering Latent Passions

Retirement can be a time to rediscover long-forgotten hobbies or explore new areas of interest that you've always wanted to pursue. This may involve:

a. Revisiting creative pursuits, such as painting, woodworking, or playing a musical instrument

b. Engaging in physical activities, like hiking, cycling, or learning a new sport

   c. Indulging in intellectual or educational interests, such as taking classes, reading, or learning a new language

   d. Exploring volunteer opportunities or community service that align with your values and skills

By tapping into your latent passions and interests, you can unlock a renewed sense of excitement and personal growth in your retirement years.

2. Expanding Social Connections

   Retirement can also provide opportunities to expand your social connections and engage in new social activities. This may include:

a. Joining clubs, organizations, or interest-based groups to connect with like-minded individuals

   b. Participating in community events, classes, or volunteer initiatives to meet new people and contribute to your local area

   c. Traveling and exploring new destinations, either independently or through organized group trips

   d. Fostering intergenerational relationships, such as mentoring younger individuals or spending time with grandchildren

By proactively building and nurturing your social network, you can combat feelings of isolation, maintain a sense of purpose, and enhance your overall well-being.

3. Embracing a Balanced Lifestyle

   Retirement offers the chance to cultivate a more balanced and fulfilling lifestyle, free from the demands of full-time employment. This may involve:

a. Prioritizing self-care activities, such as regular exercise, healthy eating, and stress management practices

   b. Dedicating time to personal interests, hobbies, and leisure pursuits

c. Maintaining a sense of structure and routine, while also allowing for flexibility and spontaneity

d. Striking a balanced approach to caregiving responsibilities, if applicable, to avoid burnout

By embracing a well-rounded retirement lifestyle, you can ensure that you maintain physical, mental, and emotional vitality throughout your later years.

Managing Finances and Healthcare in Retirement

Ensuring financial security and managing healthcare needs are critical components of a successful and fulfilling retirement. By proactively addressing these practical considerations, men over 50 can create a solid foundation for their later years.

1. Developing a Comprehensive Financial Plan

Retirement financial planning involves more than just saving and investing for the future. It encompasses a range of strategies and considerations, including:

a. Reviewing and optimizing retirement income sources, such as pensions, Social Security, and investments

b. Forecasting and planning for healthcare costs, including Medicare, supplemental insurance, and potential long-term care needs

c. Developing a sustainable withdrawal strategy from retirement accounts to ensure long-term financial stability

d. Exploring estate planning, including the creation of wills, trusts, and power of attorney documents

Collaborating with a qualified financial advisor can help ensure that your retirement finances are well-organized and positioned for long-term security and growth.

2. Navigating the Healthcare Landscape

As men transition into retirement, managing their healthcare needs becomes increasingly crucial. Key considerations include:

a. Enrolling in Medicare and understanding the various coverage options and supplemental plans

b. Identifying and establishing relationships with healthcare providers, including primary care physicians, specialists, and dentists

c. Developing a proactive approach to preventive care, screening tests, and chronic condition management

d. Exploring long-term care planning options, such as long-term care insurance or assisted living facilities, if needed

By taking a proactive and organized approach to healthcare management, retirees can ensure that their medical needs are met and their overall well-being is prioritized.

3. Maintaining Work-Life Balance and Flexibility

For some men, the transition to retirement may involve a more gradual or phased approach, where they maintain some level of paid employment or volunteer work. Strategies for managing this transition may include:

a. Exploring part-time or consulting opportunities that align with your interests and skills

b. Volunteering or engaging in community service to maintain a sense of purpose and contribution

c. Carefully balancing work commitments with personal time, leisure activities, and self-care

d. Regularly re-evaluating your work-life balance and making adjustments as needed

By maintaining a flexible and balanced approach, individuals can enjoy the benefits of retirement while also fulfilling a sense of purpose and staying engaged with the workforce.

Integrating Retirement Planning into a Holistic Wellness Approach

Retirement planning is not a standalone endeavor; it is a crucial component of a comprehensive, holistic approach to well-being in the later stages of life. By integrating retirement considerations into a broader wellness strategy, men over 50 can create a cohesive and synergistic plan for a fulfilling and empowered retirement.

1. Aligning Retirement Goals with Overall Well-Being
   When developing a retirement plan, it is essential to ensure that the financial, healthcare, and lifestyle aspects are aligned with the individual's overall health and wellness goals. This may involve:

a. Identifying the specific physical, emotional, and social needs that must be addressed during retirement
   b. Determining how the retirement plan can support the maintenance of physical function, cognitive health, and emotional well-being
   c. Integrating the various elements of the retirement plan, such as financial management, healthcare, and leisure activities, into a cohesive and balanced strategy

2. Fostering Collaborative Partnerships
   Building strong, collaborative partnerships with professionals, such as financial advisors, healthcare providers, and retirement planning specialists, is crucial for the successful integration of retirement planning into a holistic wellness approach. This may include:

a. Encouraging open communication and shared decision-making between individuals and their professional team
   b. Facilitating the coordination of services and the alignment of retirement plans with overall health and wellness goals

c. Empowering individuals to actively participate in the planning process and advocate for their needs and preferences

3. Addressing Interconnected Aspects of Well-Being

Retirement planning should not be viewed in isolation; it should be integrated with other key aspects of well-being, including physical health, emotional resilience, social connections, and cognitive function. Strategies may involve:

a. Ensuring that the retirement plan supports the maintenance of physical activity, a balanced diet, and overall physical function

b. Incorporating emotional well-being and stress management techniques into the retirement lifestyle

c. Fostering social engagement, community involvement, and the cultivation of meaningful relationships

d. Promoting cognitive stimulation, lifelong learning, and the preservation of mental acuity

4. Continuous Monitoring and Adaptation

Regularly reviewing and adapting the retirement plan is essential to ensure that it remains relevant, effective, and aligned with the individual's evolving needs and preferences. This may include:

a. Monitoring the individual's progress, identifying any changes in needs or preferences, and making adjustments accordingly

b. Staying up-to-date with the evolving landscape of retirement planning, healthcare, and community resources, and incorporating new options as they become available

c. Fostering a collaborative partnership with professionals and support networks to ensure a coordinated and responsive approach to the individual's well-being

By integrating retirement planning into a comprehensive, holistic wellness approach, men over 50 can create a robust and adaptable framework for a fulfilling, empowered, and purposeful later life.

Embracing the Journey of Retirement with Resilience and Purpose

The retirement years present a unique opportunity for men over 50 to redefine their priorities, explore new possibilities, and cultivate a sense of purpose and fulfillment. While the transition to retirement can be both exciting and daunting, embracing a proactive, comprehensive, and holistic approach can help ensure a successful and rewarding journey.

Remember, the choices and strategies you implement today can have a profound impact on your future. By prioritizing the practical, emotional, and psychological aspects of retirement planning, and integrating these elements into a broader wellness strategy, you can create a solid foundation for a fulfilling and empowered later life.

Embrace the journey of retirement with resilience and purpose, collaborate with a network of supportive professionals and communities, and trust that the steps you take will pave the way for a future filled with personal growth, adventure, and a deep sense of well-being. Your retirement is a precious chapter in your life, and the rewards it can bring are truly invaluable.

CONCLUSION

Embracing the Next Chapter with Confidence and Purpose

As you've journeyed through the pages of this comprehensive guide, you've gained invaluable insights and strategies to navigate the unique health challenges that come with aging. From preserving cardiovascular wellness and maintaining strong musculoskeletal function to addressing hormonal changes and safeguarding cognitive abilities, this book has equipped you with the knowledge and tools to take charge of your well-being in the second half of life.

However, this guide is not merely a collection of healthcare recommendations; it is a roadmap for embracing the next chapter of your life with confidence, resilience, and a profound sense of purpose. By adopting a holistic, proactive approach to your health and well-being, you can unlock a future filled with vitality, fulfillment, and the freedom to pursue the activities, relationships, and experiences that truly matter to you.

The Power of Positive Aging

Throughout this book, we've emphasized the importance of cultivating a positive mindset when it comes to the aging process. Far too often, men are bombarded with negative stereotypes and societal perceptions that portray growing older as a time of decline, limitations, and diminished capabilities. However, we firmly believe that the second half of life can be the most rewarding and empowering stage yet.

By embracing the journey of positive aging, you can redefine the narrative and unlock a renewed sense of purpose, personal growth, and the ability to thrive in the face of the unique challenges that come with growing older. This mindset shift is not just about managing physical health conditions; it's about celebrating the wisdom, experiences, and the wealth of knowledge you've accumulated over the years.

As you enter this next chapter, strive to view aging not as a burden, but as an opportunity to reinvent yourself, explore new passions, and continue making meaningful contributions to the world around you. Cultivate a deep sense of gratitude for the life you've lived and the lessons you've learned, and let these serve as the foundation for a fulfilling and empowered future.

Prioritizing Holistic Well-Being

At the heart of this guide lies a fundamental belief: that true health and wellness encompass far more than just the physical aspects of our being. By adopting a holistic approach that addresses the interconnected domains of our lives, we can create a synergistic and sustainable plan for optimal well-being in the later stages of life.

As you've discovered throughout this book, maintaining cardiovascular health, preserving musculoskeletal strength, managing hormonal changes, and safeguarding cognitive function are all crucial components of a comprehensive wellness strategy. However, these physical aspects are deeply intertwined with our emotional, mental, and social well-being.

By integrating the various facets of your health – from nutrition and exercise to stress management, emotional resilience, and community engagement – you can unlock a profound sense of balance, vitality, and the ability to thrive in the face of the changes and challenges that come with aging. This holistic approach empowers you to take a proactive, adaptable, and personalized stance towards your overall well-being, ensuring that you can continue living a life of purpose, fulfillment, and independence.

Embracing Change and Adaptability

One of the key themes that has emerged throughout this guide is the importance of embracing change and cultivating adaptability as you navigate the aging process. The human body, mind, and life circumstances are constantly evolving, and the ability to adapt to these changes is essential for maintaining a high quality of life.

Whether it's adjusting your exercise routine to accommodate physical limitations, modifying your diet to address shifting nutritional needs, or finding new ways to stay socially engaged as your relationships and roles evolve, adaptability is the cornerstone of successful aging. By approaching these changes with a flexible, resilient mindset, you can overcome obstacles, seize new opportunities, and continue to grow and thrive in the years to come.

Equally important is the willingness to continuously monitor your health, regularly reassess your needs, and make adjustments to your wellness plan as necessary. As your body, lifestyle, and priorities shift over time, your healthcare and self-care strategies must also evolve to ensure that you are always addressing your unique, ever-changing requirements.

Remember, the path to optimal health and well-being is not a linear one; it is a dynamic, lifelong journey filled with both challenges and joys. Embracing change and adaptability will not only help you navigate this journey with greater ease, but it will also empower you to capitalize on the endless possibilities that lie ahead.

The Importance of Community and Collaboration

Throughout this guide, we've emphasized the vital role that community and collaboration play in supporting men's health and well-being in the later stages of life. From building a strong network of healthcare providers to accessing community resources and fostering meaningful social connections, the power of interdependence cannot be overstated.

As you embark on this next chapter, remember that you are not alone. By actively engaging with a diverse array of healthcare professionals, support networks, and like-minded individuals, you can leverage the collective wisdom, resources, and expertise to enhance your overall well-being. Whether it's collaborating with your primary care physician to develop a personalized care plan, joining a local support group to combat feelings of isolation, or tapping into community programs that promote physical activity and social engagement, these connections can serve as a invaluable source of support, guidance, and inspiration.

Moreover, by fostering a spirit of partnership and shared decision-making with your healthcare team, you can take a more active and empowered role in your own care. This collaborative approach not only ensures that your unique needs and preferences are addressed, but it also strengthens the bond between you and your providers, leading to better health outcomes and a greater sense of trust and confidence in the healthcare system.

As you navigate the complexities of aging, remember that you do not have to go it alone. Embrace the power of community, leverage the expertise and support of those around you, and let these connections be a driving force in your journey towards optimal health and well-being.

A Call to Action: Invest in Your Future

As you reach the end of this comprehensive guide, we hope that you feel empowered, inspired, and ready to take the next steps in your journey towards a fulfilling, vibrant, and purposeful later life. The choices you make today, the habits you cultivate, and the mindset you adopt will have a profound impact on the quality of your tomorrows.

This book has provided you with a wealth of information, strategies, and practical guidance to help you navigate the unique health challenges of aging. But now, the ball is in your court. We invite you to take this knowledge, internalize the key lessons, and transform them into concrete actions that will serve as the foundation for your optimal well-being.

Whether it's committing to a balanced, nutrient-dense diet, incorporating regular physical activity into your routine, or prioritizing stress management and emotional resilience, each step you take today is an investment in your future. By embracing a proactive, holistic, and adaptable approach to your health, you are not only safeguarding your physical well-being, but you are also unlocking a renewed sense of purpose, vitality, and the freedom to fully engage in the activities, relationships, and experiences that bring you joy and fulfillment.

Remember, the journey of aging is not something to be feared or endured, but rather, an opportunity to redefine your priorities, explore new possibilities, and continue making meaningful contributions to the world around you. Embrace this next chapter with confidence, resilience, and a deep sense of purpose, and trust that the steps you take today will pave the way for a future filled with vitality, independence, and the ability to thrive in the face of life's inevitable changes.

Your well-being is a precious gift, and the time to invest in it is now. Embark on this journey with enthusiasm, curiosity, and a commitment to continuous growth and adaptation. The rewards you reap will be immeasurable, and the legacy you leave will inspire generations to come.